Advances in Paediatric Spine Surgery

Advances in Paediatric Spine Surgery

Editors

Federico Solla
Luigi Aurelio Nasto

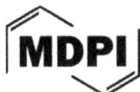 Basel • Beijing • Wuhan • Barcelona • Belgrade • Novi Sad • Cluj • Manchester

Editors
Federico Solla
Ortopaedic Surgery
University of Nice
Nice
France

Luigi Aurelio Nasto
Orthopaedic Surgery
"L. Vanvitelli" University
Hospital in Naples
Naples
Italy

Editorial Office
MDPI
St. Alban-Anlage 66
4052 Basel, Switzerland

This is a reprint of articles from the Special Issue published online in the open access journal *Children* (ISSN 2227-9067) (available at: www.mdpi.com/journal/children/special_issues/M6XM8PN6E9).

For citation purposes, cite each article independently as indicated on the article page online and as indicated below:

Lastname, A.A.; Lastname, B.B. Article Title. *Journal Name* **Year**, *Volume Number*, Page Range.

ISBN 978-3-7258-1336-0 (Hbk)
ISBN 978-3-7258-1335-3 (PDF)
doi.org/10.3390/books978-3-7258-1335-3

© 2024 by the authors. Articles in this book are Open Access and distributed under the Creative Commons Attribution (CC BY) license. The book as a whole is distributed by MDPI under the terms and conditions of the Creative Commons Attribution-NonCommercial-NoDerivs (CC BY-NC-ND) license.

Contents

About the Editors vii

Preface ix

Mathilde Gaumé, Elie Saghbiny, Lou Richard, Clélia Thouement, Raphaël Vialle and Lotfi Miladi
Pelvic Fixation Technique Using the Ilio-Sacral Screw for 173 Neuromuscular Scoliosis Patients
Reprinted from: *Children* 2024, 11, 199, doi:10.3390/children11020199 1

Federico Solla, Brice Ilharreborde, Jean-Luc Clément, Emma O. Rose, Marco Monticone, Carlo M. Bertoncelli, et al.
Patient-Specific Surgical Correction of Adolescent Idiopathic Scoliosis: A Systematic Review
Reprinted from: *Children* 2024, 11, 106, doi:10.3390/children11010106 12

Jean-Damien Metaizeau and Delphy Denis
Posterior Vertebral Body Tethering: A Preliminary Study of a New Technique to Correct Lenke 5C Lumbar Curves in Adolescent Idiopathic Scoliosis
Reprinted from: *Children* 2024, 11, 157, doi:10.3390/children11020157 31

Sławomir Zacha, Katarzyna Kotrych, Wojciech Zacha, Jowita Biernawska, Arkadiusz Ali, Dawid Ciechanowicz, et al.
Clinical Consequences of Unreconstructed Pelvic Defect Caused by Osteosarcoma with Subsequent Progressive Scoliosis in a Pediatric Patient—Case Report
Reprinted from: *Children* 2024, 11, 607, doi:10.3390/children11050607 42

Cesare Faldini, Giovanni Viroli, Matteo Traversari, Marco Manzetti, Marco Ialuna, Francesco Sartini, et al.
Ponte Osteotomies in the Surgical Treatment of Adolescent Idiopathic Scoliosis: A Systematic Review of the Literature and Meta-Analysis of Comparative Studies
Reprinted from: *Children* 2024, 11, 92, doi:10.3390/children11010092 52

Giuseppe Barone, Fabrizio Giudici, Francesco Manzini, Pierluigi Pironti, Marco Viganò, Leone Minoia, et al.
Adolescent Idiopathic Scoliosis Surgery: Postoperative Functional Outcomes at 32 Years Mean Follow-Up
Reprinted from: *Children* 2024, 11, 52, doi:10.3390/children11010052 71

Louis Boissiere, Anouar Bourghli, Fernando Guevara-Villazon, Ferran Pellisé, Ahmet Alanay, Frank Kleinstück, et al.
Rod Angulation Relationship with Thoracic Kyphosis after Adolescent Idiopathic Scoliosis Posterior Instrumentation
Reprinted from: *Children* 2024, 11, 29, doi:10.3390/children11010029 82

Ludmilla Bazin, Alexandre Ansorge, Tanguy Vendeuvre, Blaise Cochard, Anne Tabard-Fougère, Oscar Vazquez, et al.
Minimally Invasive Surgery for Posterior Spinal Instrumentation and Fusion in Adolescent Idiopathic Scoliosis: Current Status and Future Application
Reprinted from: *Children* 2023, 10, 1882, doi:10.3390/children10121882 92

**Aude Kerdoncuff, Patrice Henry, Roxane Compagnon, Franck Accadbled,
Jérôme Sales de Gauzy and Tristan Langlais**
Feasibility, Safety and Reliability of Surgeon-Directed Transcranial Motor Evoked Potentials Monitoring in Scoliosis Surgery
Reprinted from: *Children* **2023**, *10*, 1560, doi:10.3390/children10091560 . . . . **104**

**Jakub Miegoń, Sławomir Zacha, Karolina Skonieczna-Żydecka, Agata Wiczk-Bratkowska,
Agata Andrzejewska, Konrad Jarosz, et al.**
Optimising Intraoperative Fluid Management in Patients Treated with Adolescent Idiopathic Scoliosis—A Novel Strategy for Improving Outcomes
Reprinted from: *Children* **2023**, *10*, 1371, doi:10.3390/children10081371 . . . . **113**

About the Editors

Federico Solla

Federico Solla is currently a pediatric orthopaedic surgeon and the chair of the scoliosis program at Lenval University Hospital of Nice, France. His primary interest is in pediatric orthopaedic and scoliosis surgery. He is currently the co-director of the French Scoliosis Study Group (GES) under the aegis of the Frence Society of Spine Surgery (SFCR).

Dr. Solla earned his medical degree, Ph.D., and certificate of training in pediatric surgery from the medical school of Cagliari, Italy. He completed his training programs in orthopaedic and trauma surgery, spine surgery, and microsurgery at the University "Claude Bernard" of Lyon, France.

He has been involved in teaching since he was a clinical lecturer at the University of Lyon (2009 to 2012), was later a faculty member at the European Association of Neurosurgery Societies (2011 to 2015), and is currently an honorary reader and associate researcher at the University of Nice, France.

Since 2010, he has published more than 90 scientific articles in international journals; his main interests are scoliosis, pediatric spine, pediatric foot, machine learning methods, hand trauma, and congenital pseudarthrosis.

He is an active member of the French Society of Orthopaedic Surgery (SoFCOT) and the European Spine Society. He is also a fellow of the French Academy of Orthopaedics-Traumatology and a faculty member of the French College of Orthopaedic Surgeons.

Luigi Aurelio Nasto

Dr. Nasto is currently a consultant orthopedic surgeon and assistant professor at the "L. Vanvitelli" University Hospital in Naples, Italy. His main interests are pediatric orthopedic surgery and scoliosis. He previously worked as a pediatric spine surgeon at the "Gaslini" Hospital in Genoa and as a spine fellow in Canada and the United Kingdom. He has published more than 60 articles on the paediatric spine, trauma, and lower limb orthopaedic surgery.

Preface

The always-evolving field of pediatric spine surgery has seen tremendous advancements in recent years. Improvements in surgical planning, techniques, implants, and peri-operative pathways have greatly benefited our patients and their families. Nevertheless, there are still many questions to be answered and there is room for improvement.

Modern technologies, including vertebral body tethering (VBT), patient-specific strategy, self-growing rods, minimally invasive robotic assistance, and surgical navigation, are active areas of investigation. Similarly, enhanced recovery after surgery (ERAS) protocols as well as newer strategies for peri-operative management are promising tools to hasten recovery after surgery.

This Special Issue focuses on idiopathic and neuromuscular scoliosis surgery with a special interest in new technologies, new surgical techniques, and peri-operative management protocols.

Federico Solla and Luigi Aurelio Nasto
Editors

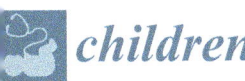

Article

Pelvic Fixation Technique Using the Ilio-Sacral Screw for 173 Neuromuscular Scoliosis Patients

Mathilde Gaumé [1,2], Elie Saghbiny [1], Lou Richard [1], Clélia Thouement [1], Raphaël Vialle [1,*] and Lotfi Miladi [2]

1. University Institute for Spine Surgery, Armand Trousseau Hospital, Sorbonne University, 26 Avenue du Dr Netter, 75012 Paris, France; mathilde.gaume@aphp.fr (M.G.); elie.saghbini@aphp.fr (E.S.); lou.richard@aphp.fr (L.R.); clelia.thouement@aphp.fr (C.T.)
2. Pediatric Orthopedic Surgery Department, Necker Hospital, APHP, University of Paris-Cité, 75015 Paris, France; l.miladi@aphp.fr
* Correspondence: raphael.vialle@aphp.fr

Abstract: Pelvic fixation remains one of the main challenging issues in non-ambulatory neuromuscular scoliosis (NMS) patients, between clinical effectiveness and a high complication rate. The objective of this multicenter and retrospective study was to evaluate the outcomes of a technique that was applied to treat 173 NMS patients. The technique is not well-known but promising; it uses the ilio-sacral screw, combined with either the posterior spinal fusion or fusionless bipolar technique, with a minimum follow-up of two years. The mean operative age of the patients was 13 ± 7 years. The mean preoperative main coronal curve was 64° and improved by a mean of −39° postoperatively. The mean preoperative pelvic obliquity was 23°, which improved by a mean of −14° postoperatively. No decrease in the frontal or sagittal correction was observed during the last follow-up. The sitting posture improved in all cases. Twenty-nine patients (17%) had a postoperative infection: twenty-six were treated with local debridement and antibiotics, and three required hardware removal. Fourteen mechanical complications (8%) occurred: screw malposition ($n = 6$), skin prominence ($n = 1$), and connector failure ($n = 1$). This type of surgery is associated with a high risk for infection. Comorbidities, rather than the surgery itself, were the main risk factors that led to complications. The ilio-sacral screw was reliable and effective in correcting pelvic obliquity in NMS patients. The introduction of intraoperative navigation should minimize the risk of screw misplacement and facilitate revision or primary fixation.

Keywords: neuromuscular scoliosis; pelvic fixation; pelvic obliquity; minimally invasive fusionless surgery; ilio-sacral screw; posterior spinal fusion

Citation: Gaumé, M.; Saghbiny, E.; Richard, L.; Thouement, C.; Vialle, R.; Miladi, L. Pelvic Fixation Technique Using the Ilio-Sacral Screw for 173 Neuromuscular Scoliosis Patients. *Children* **2024**, *11*, 199. https://doi.org/10.3390/children11020199

Academic Editors: Luigi Aurelio Nasto and Reinald Brunner

Received: 3 January 2024
Revised: 1 February 2024
Accepted: 2 February 2024
Published: 4 February 2024

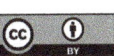

Copyright: © 2024 by the authors. Licensee MDPI, Basel, Switzerland. This article is an open access article distributed under the terms and conditions of the Creative Commons Attribution (CC BY) license (https://creativecommons.org/licenses/by/4.0/).

1. Introduction

Scoliosis is a deformity in all three planes of the spine that can occur at any stage of life. It may be idiopathic, secondary, or degenerative. Neuromuscular scoliosis can occur in patients with any type of pre-existing neuromuscular diagnosis; it is characterized by rapid worsening during growth and may continue to progress after skeletal maturity [1]. Neuromuscular scoliosis can be caused by a disorder of the brain, central or peripheral motor neurons, or muscular system. Intellectual disability and digestive, cardiac, and respiratory problems can also be associated with neuromuscular diseases. Fixed pelvic obliquity, defined as an angulation of the pelvis relative to the horizontal axis in the frontal plane, is frequently associated with spinal deformity and can lead to difficulties in maintaining a good sitting position, the onset of pain while sitting, and skin breakdown [2,3]. Conservative treatment with bracing and serial casting is poorly tolerated and has been proven to be limited [4,5]. As a result, surgery becomes necessary very quickly, with the aim to obtain a stable, compensated spine, with a balanced trunk control level [6,7]. The long posterior spinal fusion technique, using pedicular screws, or minimally invasive fusionless surgery [8], are currently the two main surgical options. Posterior vertebral arthrodesis is the gold standard of treatment for neuromuscular scoliosis, but this surgery requires skeletal maturity and is unsatisfactory before puberty [9]. In younger children, growth-sparing surgery has been developed to stabilize the spine while preserving the growth of the spine and of the thoracic cage, and postponing arthrodesis. Minimally invasive fusionless surgery is an original growth-sparing technique based on a bipolar telescopic construction whose main strength is not only to preserve spinal and thoracic growth but also to avoid arthrodesis at skeletal maturity [10].

In non-ambulatory patients, pelvic fixation is performed to achieve coronal and sagittal alignment in cases of pelvic obliquity greater than 15° or in cases of low lumbar curvature [11]. However, pelvic fixation in neuromuscular patients increases the technical difficulties and the risk of both pseudarthrosis and skin breakdown, because of their very fragile general condition and poor bone quality. These patients require multidisciplinary care in a specialized center to ensure that the procedure is planned after respiratory, nutritional, and orthopedic preparation. The difficulty in finding the best option is reflected in the wide variety of pelvic fixations described in the literature [12–15]. Modern pelvic fixation techniques include sacral, iliac, sacral alar iliac, and ilio-sacral screws. All these types of fixation techniques have their advantages and disadvantages, but what they have in common is that they all have many mechanical complications.

The ilio-sacral screw was introduced as one of Cotrel–Dubousset sacral instruments, which also include alar staples and sacral screws [16], owing to the design of a double connector by Jacques Beurier. Pelvic fixation improves the corrective lever arm and bony purchase by extending to the S1 pedicle through the two cortices of the posterior ilium [17] (Figure 1). This technique has been proven to be effective in retrospective and prospective neuromuscular scoliosis studies, with a high rate of pelvic obliquity correction (from 39.1 to 84%) and reduced rates of lumbosacral pseudarthrosis (0–0.65%) [18,19].

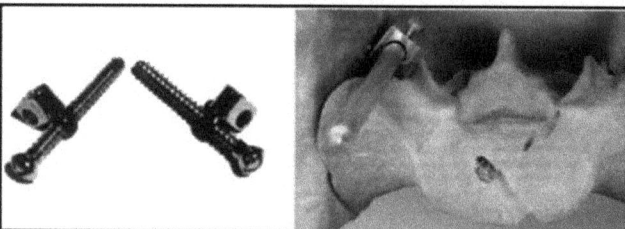

Figure 1. The ilio-sacral screw with the connector.

The objective of the following study was to validate the reliability of the ilio-sacral screw pelvic fixation technique using either posterior spinal fusion or minimally invasive fusionless surgery in a large series of neuromuscular scoliosis patients.

2. Materials and Methods

2.1. Population

A retrospective review of all consecutive non-ambulatory patients with neuromuscular scoliosis who underwent either posterior spinal fusion or minimally invasive fusionless surgery with a minimum follow-up of 2 years was conducted, including 173 patients in two academic children's hospitals (Paris, France), which are also referral centers for neuromuscular disorders. Patients who were diagnosed with neuromuscular scoliosis associated with pelvic obliquity >15° and requiring major surgery extending to the pelvis with fixation by the ilio-sacral screw were included. Patients were excluded if the scoliosis was not of neuromuscular origin or if prior spinal surgery or pelvic fixation was performed.

2.2. Operative Techniques

Patients whose triradiate cartilage was still open underwent minimally invasive fusionless surgery (minimally invasive fusionless surgery group, Figures 2 and 3), and those in whom it was fused were managed using posterior spinal fusion (posterior spinal fusion group, Figure 4).

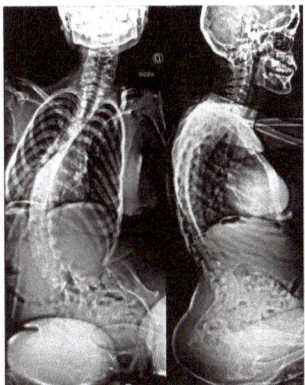
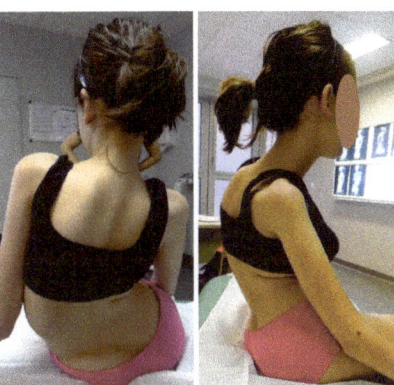

Figure 2. Preoperative X-rays and clinical pictures of a SMA2 patient.

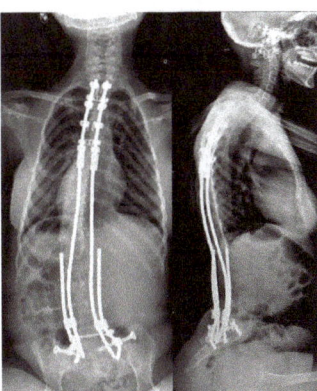
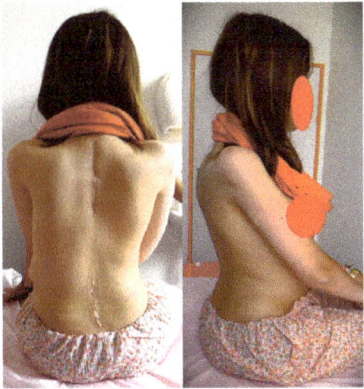

Figure 3. Postoperative X-rays and clinical pictures of the same patient, after minimally invasive fusionless surgery.

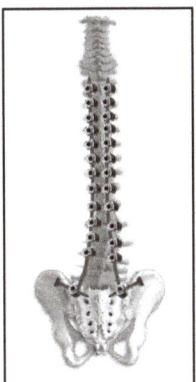

Figure 4. Posterior spinal fusion with ilio-sacral screws.

Spinal surgery was performed by the same senior surgeon for all minimally invasive fusionless surgeries (Lotfi Miladi) and all posterior spinal fusion patients (Raphael Vialle). The patient was placed in the prone position in all cases.

Posterior spinal fusion was performed using a posterior approach with spinal correction and fusion using pedicle screws, pedicle hooks, and transverse hooks at the first proximal thoracic level. The surgical technique used for the placement of the ilio-sacral screw in posterior spinal fusion procedures has been described by Zahi et al. [18]. The ilio-sacral screws were connected to the two short rods. Frontal pelvic obliquity was corrected using distraction and contraction maneuvers between the long and short rods (Figure 5).

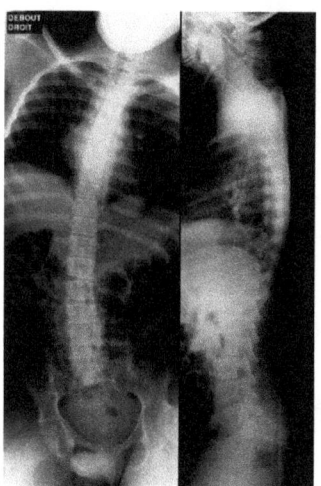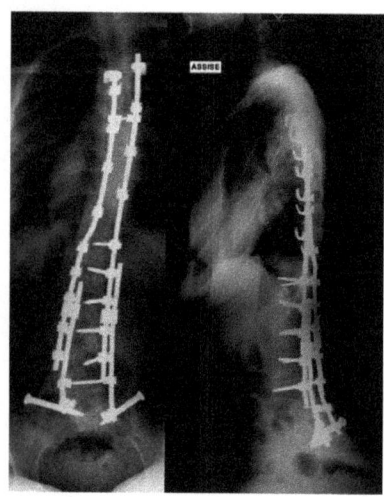

Figure 5. Pre- and postoperative X-rays after posterior spinal fusion.

The minimally invasive fusionless surgery was performed with two small midline skin incisions: the first was centered on the upper thoracic spine, and the second was centered on the lumbosacral junction. Proximal bilateral fixation was achieved at the first thoracic vertebrae using a double claw of the supralaminar and pedicle hooks attached to two adjacent vertebrae and separated by a free vertebra. A rod system composed of two long pre-curved rods was inserted intramuscularly from the proximal incision to the distal incision and attached to the proximal hooks. These rods were retained medially and attached using a side-to-side closed connector to an overlapping shorter lateral rod attached to the distal multiaxial connector of the ilio-sacral screw at S1. The amount of overlap between the two rods corresponded to the required lengthening potential of the construct. To create the final stable frame construct, cross-links were used proximally and distally.

The surgical technique used for placement of the ilio-sacral screw in minimally invasive fusionless surgery has been described by Miladi et al. [8]. The Wiltse approach allows for access to the lumbosacral joint after a short midline lumbo-pelvic incision. The posterior sacral cortex is exposed medially from the L5–S1 joint to the sacral ala, laterally and distally from the first posterior sacral foramina. A trough was made lateral to the L5–S1 joint and above the first posterior sacral foramen. The ilio-sacral connector was fixed using a connector holder and inserted into the trough. A guide was attached to the connector holder to facilitate screw insertion. Once the guide was removed, the cannulated screw was inserted percutaneously through the ilio-sacral connector from the posterior part of the iliac wing towards the sacrum to reach the body of S1. The screw was then locked within the ilio-sacral connectors.

The screw length can vary. The sizes were selected based on the anatomical parameters of the preoperative films. Fully threaded ilio-sacral screws were implanted freehand.

Postoperative management was performed for a few days in the intensive care unit, followed by management in a traditional orthopedic ward. Rehabilitation was performed at home or at a rehabilitation center.

2.3. Outcomes Assessment

Age and etiology of the neuromuscular disorder were recorded as demographic data.

Radiographs were obtained in the sitting position before surgery, after surgery, and at the last follow-up [20]. Measurements were obtained using PACS-Carestream software 12.0 (Rochester, NY, USA: Carestream Health). The Cobb angle of the main curve and pelvic obliquity were measured. The Cobb angle was measured by drawing lines parallel to the upper border of the upper vertebral body and the lower border of the lowest vertebra of the structural curve, and then by drawing perpendicular lines from these lines to cross each other. Pelvic obliquity was defined as "the angle subtended by a line drawn between the most proximal points of the iliac crest and a line drawn parallel to the lower end of the roentgenogram" [21].

Complications including surgical site infections and the mechanical failure of the ilio-sacral screw were recorded.

Patients and/or caregiver-reported outcome questionnaires were also used to assess sitting posture (same, better, or worse) and comfort improvement (same, better, or worse). Pain was rated from 0 to 10, with 0 indicating the absence of pain and 10 indicating the maximum pain.

2.4. Statistics

Data were processed using SPSS V23 software (IBM Corporation, Armonk, NY, USA). Comparisons between the two groups were performed using Fisher's exact test or the chi-squared test. A comparison of deformity correction was performed using a non-parametric analysis of paired samples. Statistical significance was set at $p < 0.05$.

3. Results

3.1. Demographic Data

A total of 173 patients were included, and none were lost to follow-up. Posterior spinal fusion was performed in 62 patients and minimally invasive fusionless surgery was performed in 111 patients. All patients were non-ambulatory. The mean operative age was 13.7 ± 7 years (12 in the minimally invasive fusionless surgery group and 15 in the posterior spinal fusion group). The etiologies included cerebral palsy ($n = 113$), spinal muscular atrophy ($n = 19$), muscular dystrophy ($n = 14$), flaccid paraplegia ($n = 11$), myelomeningocele ($n = 9$), and Rett syndrome ($n = 7$). Significantly more patients had cerebral palsy and myelomeningocele in the minimally invasive fusionless surgery group ($p < 0.05$).

3.2. Radiological Data

The differences between the main curve deformity and pelvic obliquity for both groups preoperatively and at the latest follow-up are reported in Table 1. The preoperative major curve was higher in the minimally invasive fusionless surgery group (77.0 vs. 50.5°). Preoperative pelvic obliquity was not significantly greater in the two groups. Before surgical correction, the mean Cobb angle of the main coronal curve was 63.8°, which improved by a mean of −39.5° (−60%) postoperatively. Mean preoperative pelvic obliquity was 23.0°, which improved by a mean of −14° postoperatively (61%). Pelvic obliquity was better corrected in the minimally invasive fusionless surgery group. No loss of frontal or sagittal correction was observed at the last follow-up.

Table 1. Main demographic data and radiologic outcomes of the series.

	PSF	MIFS	PSF and MIFS	p
Patients, n	62	111	173	
Mean age, years	15 (12 to 19)	12 (6 to 19)	13.7 (6 to 19)	
Etiology				
Muscular dystrophy, n	4 (6.5%)	10	14	0.0554
Cerebral palsy, n	42 (67.7%)	71	102	0.617
Flaccid Paraplegia, n	7 (11.3%)	4	11	0.057
Spinal muscular atrophy, n	6 (9.7%)	13	19	0.681
Rett syndrom, n	2 (3.2%)	5	7	1
Myelomeningocele	1 (1.6%)	8	9	0.159
Infections, n	13 (21%)	16 (14.4%)	29 (16.7%)	0.02 *
Local debridment and antibiotics, n	12	14	26	
Hardware removal, n	1	2	3	
Mechanical complications, n	5 (8.1%)	9 (8.1%)	14 (8%)	0.091
Early mobilization of S1 screw, n	5	1	6	
S1 root irritation, n	0	6	6	
Connector failure, n	0	1	1	
Ilio-sacral screw skin prominence, n	0	1	1	
Preoperative pelvic obliquity, (°), mean	23	23	23	
Last FU pelvic obliquity improvement (°), mean	−10.2 (44%)	−17.8 (77%)	−14	
Preoperative Cobb angle, (°), mean	50.5	77	63.8	
Last FU Cobb correction improvement, (°), mean	−31.1 (61%)	−47.8 (62%)	−39.5	
Loss of frontal or sagittal correction	None	None	None	
Sitting posture and comfort improvement	All cases	All cases	All cases	

PSF = posterior spinal fusion; MIFS = minimally invasive fusionless surgery; FU = follow-up; * Statistically significant.

3.3. Complications

Fourteen mechanical complications (8%) occurred: the early mobilization of one ilio-sacral screw made it necessary to change the screw for a longer one percutaneously ($n = 6$); screw malposition with S1 root irritation ($n = 6$); screw skin prominence ($n = 1$); and connector failure ($n = 1$). There were no significant differences in mechanical complications between the minimally invasive fusionless surgery and posterior spinal fusion groups.

Twenty-nine patients (17%) had an early postoperative infection, with favorable outcomes in the 26 patients who were treated with local wound debridement and antibiotics. In three cases, a persistent chronic Staphylococcus aureus infection required hardware removal. The outcome was favorable in all patients, with satisfactory healing and no recurrence of infection following hardware removal. On average, the patients waited one year before being re-instrumented.

3.4. Quality of Life

According to the patients and/or caregivers, sitting posture and comfort were qualified as "better" in all cases after surgery, with a clear improvement in transfers in daily life, particularly from bed to chair.

The only patients who described postoperative pain were due to S1 nerve root irritation, associated with ilio-sacral screw malposition. The pain was relieved once the screw path was corrected.

4. Discussion

This study focused on the outcomes of patients with neuromuscular scoliosis who underwent either posterior spinal fusion or minimally invasive fusionless surgery with pelvic extension using ilio-sacral screws. This is the largest series described in the literature that compares ilio-sacral screws in the same cohort. The results demonstrate that fixation using ilio-sacral screw is effective in pediatric patients with neuromuscular scoliosis, with a 60% correction of the Cobb angle and a 61% correction of pelvic obliquity, respectively. Pelvic obliquity correction was better in the minimally invasive fusionless surgery group than in the posterior spinal fusion group because of repetitive surgeries for lengthening procedures in cases of major residual pelvic deformity [8]. The lengthening procedure was performed with a previous distal incision for access to the side-to-side connectors and the possibility of the asymmetrical lengthening of the rods.

The present results are consistent with the current literature, with a 77% correction of pelvic obliquity and a 52% correction of the Cobb angle in a consecutive series of 167 neuromuscular scoliosis patients who exclusively underwent minimally invasive fusionless surgery with ilio-sacral screw pelvic fixation. Sixteen mechanical complications in nine patients happened: screw prominence ($n = 1$), connector failure ($n = 4$), and screw malposition ($n = 11$). Unplanned surgery was required in seven cases; two cases were managed during rod lengthening, and seven did not require treatment [22]. Miladi et al. [17] reported a correction of the Cobb angle of the main curve ranging from 53% to 70%, and the correction of pelvic obliquity ranging from 60% to 84%, in a series of 154 patients with neuromuscular scoliosis who underwent posterior spinal fusion with the ilio-sacral screw. Twenty-five complications were observed in seven patients, including four dislodgments of the ilio-sacral screw. The complications were caused by an infection in three patients and by a failure to check the tightness of the screw in one patient. Lumbosacral pseudarthrosis occurred in one patient, whereas none were reported in our series. In the literature, the pseudarthrosis rate in neuromuscular scoliosis patients ranges from 1.8 to 15% [23–25].

The literature on adult spinal deformity provides further insight into the effects of pelvic fixation with ilio-sacral screws in neuromuscular scoliosis patients. Wolff et al. [26] examined the outcomes in 15 adults with neuromuscular scoliosis who underwent minimally invasive fusionless surgery from the thoracic spine to the pelvis. Significant improvements in pain and balance were reported in all the patients. Only one connector failure was reported because of an inappropriate choice of the implant, which was too small (pediatric instead of adult shape).

The correction rate was also comparable to that of other pelvic fixation options, with a 63% mean correction of the Cobb angle of the main curve, and a 55% mean correction of pelvic obliquity with the sacral alar iliac fixation technique reported in the series by Jain et al. [27]. Sponseller et al. [28] compared the two-year postoperative radiographic parameters of 32 pediatric patients who underwent the procedure with the sacral alar iliac fixation technique and 27 patients who underwent the procedure with the sacroiliac technique. Among the patients who received the procedure with the sacral alar iliac fixation technique, the mean correction of pelvic obliquity was 70% and the mean Cobb angle correction was 67%. Among the patients who received the procedure using the sacroiliac technique, the values were 50% and 60%, respectively. Compared with other traditional techniques, sacral alar iliac screws provided a significantly better correction of pelvic obliquity, but no difference in the Cobb angle correction of the main curve or complications were observed.

We observed a rather high infection rate of 17%, which, however, seems to be within the range of previous reports in the literature (from 6 to 20%) [29,30]. Surgical site infections were more frequent in the minimally invasive fusionless surgery group than in the posterior spinal fusion group. The surgical approach may not influence the incidence of infection. For example, the correction of pelvic obliquity using the "T construct" for pelvic fixation requires an extensive dissection of the tissue at the caudal end of the spine to insert the horizontal portion of the "T", with a similar infection rate of 18% in a series of 60 neuromuscular scoliosis patients [31]. Due to poor nutrition, poor wound healing, incontinence, and impaired communication, neuromuscular scoliosis procedures are known to be associated with frequent postoperative infections [32–34]. The incidence of infection in the minimally invasive fusionless surgery group may also be related to the possibility of iterative rod lengthening, with an increased infection risk after each procedure. The advent of one-way self-expanding rods, which are designed to avoid repeated surgery due to their free rod-sliding capabilities, should reduce the surgical site infection rate of minimally invasive fusionless surgeries in further studies. The infection rate decreased to 9% in a preliminary report of a prospective series of 21 patients who underwent procedures using one-way self-expanding rods with distal fixation using ilio-sacral screws after a minimum follow-up of three years. No complications related to the ilio-sacral screws have been reported [35].

In the present study, the mechanical complication rate was 8%, which is consistent with other types of pelvic fixation procedures in the literature. Procedures using the S2 alar iliac screw fixation technique have a 4 to 7% implant failure rate, and similar revision rates for implant failure [12,36,37].

The most common complication related to the use of ilio-sacral screws in the present series was S1 root irritation due to screw malposition (3.4%), which was also the most common reason for revision. However, these malpositions occurred before systematic preoperative control using 3D CT scanning. Notably, screw loosening was observed radiographically in a few X-rays with an osteolytic zone around the ilio-sacral screw <5 mm, but with no clinical or mechanical consequences in any patient. The risk of malposition is not just a problem for ilio-sacral screws, but also for other types of pelvic fixation, with various rates across studies. In adults, the breakthrough rate of procedures using the S2 alar iliac screw was 18% [38]. In Hassan et al.'s [39] pediatric cohort of 25 patients, screw breakthrough involving the lateral iliac-wing cortex occurred in eight (32%) patients. Eight percent of the patients had screw malposition, as confirmed by a postoperative CT scan. In contrast, Sponseller et al. [28], who has promoted the S2 alar iliac screw fixation technique in the pediatric population, reported no cases of malposition.

A recent computed tomography study demonstrated the ideal ilio-sacral screw trajectory to avoid malpositioning in children with non-neuromuscular scoliosis, which differs from that in adults. The mean optimal angles were $32.3° \pm 3.6°$, $33.8° \pm 4.7°$, $30.2° \pm 5.0°$, and $30.4° \pm 4.7°$ in females < 10 years old, males < 10 years old, females > 10 years old, and males > 10 years old, respectively. The mean optimal angle differed between the two age groups ($p = 0.004$) but not between females and males ($p = 0.55$). The mean optimal screw length was 73.4 ± 9.9 mm. The transverse spinal canal anatomical parameters varied with age ($p = 0.02$) and sex in older children ($p = 0.008$), and the sagittal parameters varied with sex ($p = 0.04$) [40]. Such computed tomography studies should be of interest for patients with neuromuscular scoliosis.

Although the ilio-sacral screw technique is operator-dependent with a relatively longer learning curve than other pelvic fixation techniques, the emergence of new ancillaries should improve the accuracy of ilio-sacral screw positioning in the future. Moreover, innovative navigation methods and augmented reality surgery-like conditions could be interesting new teaching tools and surgical aids to enhance visualization and improve patient outcomes [41–43].

The ilio-sacral screw also has other strong advantages, particularly the low profile of the implant and its deep location, which permits a decrease in the risk of implant prominence and skin ulceration, which was reported in only one very skinny patient weighing <20 kg. The ilio-sacral screw can also be placed without exposing the iliac crest and without the potential devascularization of the overlying soft tissues, which may reduce complications due to implant prominence. The sacral alar iliac technique also has the key advantage of eliminating the need for subcutaneous muscle dissection over the iliac crest and decreasing the risk of implant prominence. In contrast, screw prominence reached over 11% with the iliac screw fixation technique [11].

The absence of pain in the sitting position after ilio-sacral screw surgery may be due to the screw path not crossing the sacroiliac joint and the tightening of the ilio-sacral screw perpendicular to the joint plane, allowing for a protective syndesmosis effect on the sacroiliac joint. Crossing the sacroiliac joint in childhood could lead to long-term pain, which has not yet been well evaluated, particularly with the S2 wing screw technique. Multiple pedicular screw fixation improves spinal rigidity in posterior spinal fusion constructs. Under these conditions, patients had an improved postoperative course with earlier mobilization and return to a comfortable sitting position. The improvement in spinal stabilization over time permitted a reduction in the need for a postoperative cast or brace in a minimally invasive fusionless surgery construct.

The absence of screw pullout could be due to the rod connection in the center of the screw and the perpendicular position of the screw to the iliac crest, crossing both cortices and ending transversely in the S1 body.

Our study had several limitations that should be addressed in future studies. First, it was retrospective and based on reported findings. There were no comparisons or randomized groups with other pelvic fixation techniques. It was also difficult to assess functional outcomes in our patients. This is particularly true for patients with cerebral palsy and severe intellectual disability [44]. Finally, the effect of posterior spinal fusion or minimally invasive fusionless surgery with the ilio-sacral screw pelvic fixation technique in children with ambulatory ability has not yet been evaluated. Drake et al. published the results of a large study of 118 patients with neuromuscular scoliosis, including 11 ambulatory patients with pelvic extension using either sacral alar iliac or iliac screws [45]. They found that all patients were able to walk with the same or better function after posterior spinal fusion with pelvic extension. In addition, in terms of hardware failure, no significant difference was found between the ambulatory and non-ambulatory groups.

Despite these limitations, this study is the first in the literature to evaluate the effect of ilio-sacral screw pelvic fixation in patients receiving either posterior spinal fusion or minimally invasive fusionless surgery, incorporating the most recent and relevant references in the field, and demonstrating that this fixation technique is effective in this specific population.

5. Conclusions

Despite the high rate of infectious complications (17%), the ilio-sacral screw is an effective tool to treat frontal and sagittal pelvic obliquity and spinal deformity in neuromuscular scoliosis patients. The mechanical complication rate was lower than that of other pelvic fixation procedures, as described in the literature. Intraoperative navigation should minimize the risk of nerve root injury and facilitate revision or primary fixation in patients with disturbed sacropelvic anatomy.

Author Contributions: Conceptualization, M.G., R.V. and L.M.; data curation, R.V. and L.M.; formal analysis, M.G.; investigation, M.G., R.V. and L.M.; methodology, E.S., R.V. and L.M.; resources, R.V. and L.M.; supervision, R.V. and L.M.; validation, E.S., L.R., C.T., R.V. and L.M.; visualization, E.S., L.R. and C.T.; writing—original draft, M.G.; writing—review and editing, M.G., E.S., L.R., C.T., R.V. and L.M. All authors have read and agreed to the published version of the manuscript.

Funding: This research received no external funding.

Institutional Review Board Statement: The study was conducted in accordance with the Declaration of Helsinki and approved by the Local Ethical Review Board of the MAMUTH FHU under the reference 2023-IRB-FHU-0132 (Paris, 1 December 2023).

Informed Consent Statement: Informed consent was obtained from all the subjects involved in the study. Written informed consent was obtained from the patients and/or caregivers for the publication of this paper.

Data Availability Statement: All data are available on demand from the corresponding author. The data are not publicly available because of privacy concerns.

Conflicts of Interest: The authors declare no conflicts of interest.

References

1. Thometz, J.G.; Simon, S.R. Progression of scoliosis after skeletal maturity in institutionalized adults who have cerebral palsy. *J. Bone Jt. Surg. Am.* **1988**, *70*, 1290–1296. [CrossRef]
2. Yen, W.; Gartenberg, A.; Cho, W. Pelvic obliquity associated with neuromuscular scoliosis in cerebral palsy: Cause and treatment. *Spine Deform.* **2021**, *9*, 1259–1265. [CrossRef] [PubMed]
3. Hasler, C.; Brunner, R. Spine deformities in patients with cerebral palsy; the role of the pelvis. *J. Child. Orthop.* **2020**, *14*, 9–16. [CrossRef] [PubMed]
4. Saito, N.; Ebara, S.; Ohotsuka, K.; Kumeta, H.; Takaoka, K. Natural history of scoliosis in spastic cerebral palsy. *Lancet* **1998**, *351*, 1687–1692. [CrossRef]
5. Olafsson, Y.; Saraste, H.; Al-Dabbagh, Z. Brace treatment in neuromuscular spine deformity. *J. Pediatr. Orthop.* **1999**, *19*, 376–379. [CrossRef] [PubMed]
6. Whitaker, C.; Burton, D.C.; Asher, M. Treatment of selected neuromuscular patients with posterior instrumentation and arthrodesis ending with lumbar pedicle screw anchorage. *Spine* **2000**, *25*, 2312–2318. [CrossRef]
7. Lubicky, J.P.; McCarthy, R.E. Sacral pelvic fixation in neuromuscular deformities. *Semin. Spine Surg.* **2004**, *16*, 126–133. [CrossRef]
8. Miladi, L.; Gaume, M.; Khouri, N.; Johnson, M.; Topouchian, V.; Glorion, C. Minimally invasive surgery for neuromuscular scoliosis: Results and complications in a series of one hundred patients. *Spine* **2018**, *43*, E968–E975. [CrossRef]
9. Dimeglio, A.; Canavese, F. The immature spine: Growth and idiopathic scoliosis. *Ann. Transl. Med.* **2020**, *8*, 22. [CrossRef]
10. Gaume, M.; Langlais, T.; Loiselet, K.; Pannier, S.; Skalli, W.; Vergari, C.; Miladi, L. Spontaneous induced bone fusion in minimally invasive fusionless bipolar fixation in neuromuscular scoliosis: A computed tomography analysis. *Eur. Spine J.* **2023**, *32*, 2550–2557. [CrossRef]
11. Modi, H.N.; Suh, S.W.; Song, H.-R.; Yang, J.H.; Jajodia, N. Evaluation of pelvic fixation in neuromuscular scoliosis: A retrospective study in 55 patients. *Int. Orthop.* **2010**, *34*, 89–96. [CrossRef]
12. Moon, E.S.; Nanda, A.; Park, J.O.; Moon, S.H.; Lee, H.M.; Kim, J.Y.; Yoon, S.P.; Kim, H.S. Pelvic Obliquity in Neuromuscular Scoliosis Radiologic Comparative Results of Single-Stage Posterior Versus Two-Stage Anterior and Posterior Approach. *Spine* **2011**, *36*, 146–152. [CrossRef]
13. Shabtai, L.; Andras, L.M.; Portman, M.; Harris, L.R.; Choi, P.D.; Tolo, V.T.; Skaggs, D.L. Sacral alar iliac (sacral alar iliac) screws fail 75% less frequently than iliac screws in neuromuscular scoliosis. *J. Pediatr. Orthop.* **2017**, *37*, e470–e475. [CrossRef]
14. Peelle, M.W.; Lenke, L.G.; Bridwell, K.H.; Sides, B. Comparison of pelvic fixation techniques in neuromuscular spinal deformity correction: Galveston rod versus iliac and lumbosacral screws. *Spine* **2006**, *31*, 2392–2398. [CrossRef] [PubMed]
15. Anari, J.B.; Spiegel, D.A.; Baldwin, K.D. Neuromuscular scoliosis and pelvic fixation in 2015: Where do we stand? *World J. Orthop.* **2015**, *6*, 564–566. [CrossRef] [PubMed]
16. Cotrel, Y.; Dubousset, J.; Guillaumat, M. New universal instrumentation in spinal surgery. *Clin. Orthop. Relat. Res.* **1988**, *227*, 10–23. [CrossRef] [PubMed]
17. Miladi, L.T.; Ghanem, I.B.; Draoui, M.M.; Zeller, R.D.; Dubousset, J.F. Iliosacral screw fixation for pelvic obliquity in neuromuscular scoliosis. A long-term follow-up study. *Spine* **1997**, *22*, 1722–1729. [CrossRef] [PubMed]
18. Zahi, R.; Vialle, R.; Abelin, K.; Mary, P.; Khouri, N.; Damsin, J.-P. Spinopelvic fixation with iliosacral screws in neuromuscular spinal deformities: Results in a prospective cohort of 62 patients. *Childs Nerv. Syst.* **2010**, *26*, 81–86. [CrossRef] [PubMed]
19. Neustadt, J.B.; Shufflebarger, H.L.; Cammisa, F.P. Spinal fusions to the pelvis augmented by Cotrel-Dubousset instrumentation for neuromuscular scoliosis. *J. Pediatr. Orthop.* **1992**, *12*, 465–469. [CrossRef] [PubMed]
20. Gupta, M.C.; Wijesekera, S.; Sossan, A.D.; Martin, L.; Vogel, L.C.; Boakes, J.L.; Lerman, J.A.; McDonald, C.M.; Betz, R.R. Reliability of radiographic parameters in neuromuscular scoliosis. *Spine* **2007**, *32*, 691–695. [CrossRef] [PubMed]
21. Osebold, W.R.; Mayfield, J.K.; Winter, R.B.; Moe, J.H. Surgical treatment of paralytic scoliosis associated with myelomeningocele. *J. Bone Jt. Surg Am.* **1982**, *64*, 841–856. [CrossRef]
22. Gaume, M.; Vergari, C.; Khouri, N.; Skalli, W.; Glorion, C.; Miladi, L. Minimally Invasive Surgery for Neuromuscular Scoliosis: Results and Complications at a Minimal Follow-up of 5 Years. *Spine* **2021**, *46*, 1696–1704. [CrossRef]
23. Edwards, B.T.; Zura, R.; Bertrand, S.; Leonard, S.; Pellett, J. Treatment of neuromuscular scoliosis with posterior spinal fusion using the Galveston technique: A retrospective review and results of 62 patients. *J. Long Term. Eff. Med. Implant.* **2003**, *13*, 437–444. [CrossRef] [PubMed]
24. Benson, E.R.; Thomson, J.D.; Smith, B.G.; Banta, J.V. Results and morbidity in a consecutive series of patients undergoing spinal fusion for neuromuscular scoliosis. *Spine* **1988**, *23*, 2308–2317, discussion 2318. [CrossRef] [PubMed]
25. Teli, M.; Elsebaie, H.; Biant, L.; Noordeen, H. Neuromuscular scoliosis treated by segmental third-generation instrumented spinal fusion. *J. Spinal. Disord. Tech.* **2005**, *18*, 430–438. [CrossRef] [PubMed]
26. Wolff, S.; Moreau, P.E.; Miladi, L.; Riouallon, G. Is minimally invasive bipolar technique a better alternative to long fusion for adult neuromuscular scoliosis? *Global. Spine J.* **2023**, 21925682231159347. [CrossRef]
27. Jain, A.; Sullivan, B.T.; Kuwabara, A.; Kebaish, K.M.; Sponseller, P.D. Sacral-alar-iliac fixation in children with neuromuscular scoliosis: Minimum 5-year follow-up. *World Neurosurg.* **2017**, *108*, 474–478. [CrossRef]
28. Sponseller, P.D.; Zimmerman, R.M.; Ko, P.S.; Gunne, A.F.P.T.; Mohamed, A.S.; Chang, T.-L.; Kebaish, K.M. Low profile pelvic fixation with the sacral alar iliac technique in the pediatric population improves results at two-year minimum follow-up. *Spine* **2010**, *35*, 1887–1889. [CrossRef]

29. Aleissa, S.; Parsons, D.; Grant, J.; Harder, J.; Howard, J. Deep wound infection following pediatric scoliosis surgery: Incidence and analysis of risk factors. *Can. J. Surg.* **2011**, *54*, 263–269. [CrossRef]
30. Cahill, P.J.; Warnick, D.E.; Lee, M.J.; Gaughan, J.; Vogel, L.E.; Hammerberg, K.W.; Sturm, P.F. Infection afer spinal fusion for pediatric spinal deformity: Tirty years of experience at a single institution. *Spine* **2010**, *35*, 1211–1217. [CrossRef]
31. Bouyer, B.; Bachy, M.; Zahi, R.; Thévenin-Lemoine, C.; Mary, P.; Vialle, R. Correction of pelvic obliquity in neuromuscular spinal deformities using the "T construct": Results and complications in a prospective series of 60 patients. *Eur. Spine J.* **2014**, *23*, 163–171. [CrossRef] [PubMed]
32. Ramo, B.A.; Roberts, D.W.; Tuason, D.; McClung, A.; Paraison, L.E.; Moore IV, H.G.; Sucato, D.J. Surgical site infections after posterior spinal fusion for neuromuscular scoliosis: A thirty year experience at a single institution. *J. Bone Jt. Surg. Am.* **2014**, *96*, 2038–2048. [CrossRef] [PubMed]
33. Sponseller, P.D.; LaPorte, D.M.; Hungerford, M.W.; Eck, K.; Bridwell, K.H.; Lenke, L.G. Deep wound infections after neuromuscular scoliosis surgery: A multicenter study of risk factors and treatment outcomes. *Spine* **2000**, *25*, 2461–2466. [CrossRef] [PubMed]
34. Weissmann, K.A.; Weissmann, K.A.; Lafage, V.; Lafage, V.; Pitaque, C.B.; Pitaque, C.B.; Lafage, R.; Lafage, R.; Huaiquilaf, C.M.; Huaiquilaf, C.M.; et al. Neuromuscular scoliosis: Comorbidities and complications. *Asian Spine J.* **2021**, *15*, 778–790. [CrossRef] [PubMed]
35. Gaume, M.; Hajj, R.; Khouri, N.; Johnson, M.; Miladi, L. One-Way Self-Expanding Rod in Neuromuscular Scoliosis: Preliminary Results of a Prospective Series of 21 Patients. *JBJS Open Access* **2021**, *6*, e21.00089. [CrossRef]
36. Ilyas, H.; Place, H.; Puryear, A. A comparison of early clinical and radiographic complications of iliac screw fixation versus S2 alar iliac (S2AI) fixation in the adult and pediatric populations. *J. Spinal. Disord. Tech.* **2015**, *28*, E199–E205. [CrossRef]
37. Ravindra, V.M.; Mazur, M.D.; Brockmeyer, D.L.; Kraus, K.L.; Ropper, A.E.; Hanson, D.S.; Dahl, B.T. Clinical Effectiveness of S2-Alar Iliac Screws in Spinopelvic Fixation in Pediatric Neuromuscular Scoliosis: Systematic Literature Review. *Global. Spine J.* **2020**, *10*, 1066–1074. [CrossRef]
38. Shillingford, J.N.; Laratta, J.L.; Tan, L.A.; Sarpong, N.O.; Lin, J.D.; Fischer, C.R.; Lehman, R.A.; Kim, Y.J.; Lenke, L.G. The free-hand technique for s2-alar-iliac screw placement: A safe and effective method for sacropelvic fixation in adult spinal deformity. *J. Bone Jt. Surg. Am.* **2018**, *100*, 334–342. [CrossRef]
39. Hassan, S.K.; Simon, L.; Campana, M.; Julien-Marsollier, F.; Simon, A.-L.; Ilharreborde, B. S2-Alar-iliac screw fixation for paediatric neuromuscular scoliosis: Preliminary results after two years. *Orthop. Traumatol. Surg. Res.* **2022**, *108*, 103234. [CrossRef]
40. Gaume, M.; Triki, M.A.; Glorion, C.; Breton, S.; Miladi, L. Optimal ilio-sacral screw trajectory in paediatric patients: A computed tomography study. *Acta Orthop. Belg.* **2021**, *87*, 285–291. [CrossRef]
41. Azad, T.D.; Warman, A.; Tracz, J.A.; Hughes, L.P.; Judy, B.F.; Witham, T.F. Augmented reality in spine surgery—Past, present, and future. *Spine J.* **2024**, *24*, 1–13. [CrossRef] [PubMed]
42. Asada, T.; Simon, C.Z.; Lu, A.Z.; Adida, S.; Dupont, M.; Parel, P.M.; Zhang, J.; Bhargava, S.; Morse, K.W.; Dowdell, J.E.; et al. Robot-navigated pedicle screw insertion can reduce intraoperative blood loss and length of hospital stay: Analysis of 1633 patients utilizing propensity score matching. *Spine J.* **2024**, *24*, 118–124. [CrossRef]
43. Yamout, T.; Orosz, L.D.; Good, C.R.; Jazini, E.; Allen, B.; Gum, J.L. Technological Advances in Spine Surgery: Navigation, Robotics, and Augmented Reality. *Orthop. Clin. N. Am.* **2023**, *54*, 237–246. [CrossRef]
44. Moreau, M.; Mahood, J.; Moreau, K.; Berg, D.; Hill, D.; Raso, J. Assessing the impact of pelvic obliquity in postoperative neuromuscular scoliosis. *Stud. Health Technol. Inf.* **2002**, *91*, 481–485.
45. Drake, L.; Sukkarieh, H.; McDonald, T.; Bhanat, E.; Quince, E.; Atkins, M.; Wright, P.; Brooks, J. Effect of pelvic fixation on ambulation in children with neuromuscular scoliosis. *World J. Orthop.* **2022**, *13*, 753–759. [CrossRef] [PubMed]

Disclaimer/Publisher's Note: The statements, opinions and data contained in all publications are solely those of the individual author(s) and contributor(s) and not of MDPI and/or the editor(s). MDPI and/or the editor(s) disclaim responsibility for any injury to people or property resulting from any ideas, methods, instructions or products referred to in the content.

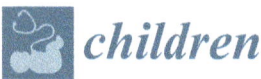

Systematic Review

Patient-Specific Surgical Correction of Adolescent Idiopathic Scoliosis: A Systematic Review

Federico Solla [1,*], Brice Ilharreborde [2], Jean-Luc Clément [1], Emma O. Rose [3], Marco Monticone [4], Carlo M. Bertoncelli [1] and Virginie Rampal [1]

1. Paediatric Orthopaedic Unit, Lenval Foundation, 57, Avenue de la Californie, 06200 Nice, France; clement.jluc@wanadoo.fr (J.-L.C.); carlo.bertoncelli@hpu.lenval.com (C.M.B.); virginie.rocher-rampal@hpu.lenval.com (V.R.)
2. Paediatric Orthopaedic Unit, Hôpital Robert Debré, AP-HP, 75019 Paris, France; brice.ilharreborde@aphp.fr
3. Krieger School of Arts & Sciences, Homewood Campus, John Hopkins University, Baltimore, MD 21218, USA
4. Department of Surgical Sciences, University of Cagliari, 09124 Cagliari, Italy; marco.monticone@unica.it
* Correspondence: federico.solla@hpu.lenval.com; Tel.: +33-4-9203-0491

Abstract: The restoration of sagittal alignment is fundamental to the surgical correction of adolescent idiopathic scoliosis (AIS). Despite established techniques, some patients present with inadequate postoperative thoracic kyphosis (TK), which may increase the risk of proximal junctional kyphosis (PJK) and imbalance. There is a lack of knowledge concerning the effectiveness of patient-specific rods (PSR) with measured sagittal curves in achieving a TK similar to that planned in AIS surgery, the factors influencing this congruence, and the incidence of PJK after PSR use. This is a systematic review of all types of studies reporting on the PSR surgical correction of AIS, including research articles, proceedings, and gray literature between 2013 and December 2023. From the 28,459 titles identified in the literature search, 81 were assessed for full-text reading, and 7 studies were selected. These included six cohort studies and a comparative study versus standard rods, six monocentric and one multicentric, three prospective and four retrospective studies, all with a scientific evidence level of 4 or 3. They reported a combined total of 355 AIS patients treated with PSR. The minimum follow-up was between 4 and 24 months. These studies all reported a good match between predicted and achieved TK, with the main difference ranging from 0 to 5 degrees, $p > 0.05$, despite the variability in surgical techniques and the rods' properties. There was no proximal junctional kyphosis, whereas the current rate from the literature is between 15 and 46% with standard rods. There are no specific complications related to PSR. The exact role of the type of implants is still unknown. The preliminary results are, therefore, encouraging and support the use of PSR in AIS surgery.

Keywords: children; thoracic spine; rods; planning; thoracic kyphosis; pre-bent; contouring

Citation: Solla, F.; Ilharreborde, B.; Clément, J.-L.; Rose, E.O.; Monticone, M.; Bertoncelli, C.M.; Rampal, V. Patient-Specific Surgical Correction of Adolescent Idiopathic Scoliosis: A Systematic Review. *Children* **2024**, *11*, 106. https://doi.org/10.3390/children11010106

Academic Editor: Syuji Takei

Received: 5 December 2023
Revised: 3 January 2024
Accepted: 11 January 2024
Published: 15 January 2024

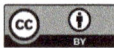

Copyright: © 2024 by the authors. Licensee MDPI, Basel, Switzerland. This article is an open access article distributed under the terms and conditions of the Creative Commons Attribution (CC BY) license (https://creativecommons.org/licenses/by/4.0/).

1. Introduction

The pathological coronal curve of adolescent idiopathic scoliosis (AIS) combined with the sagittal alignment causes a 3D deformity [1–3]. This automatically leads to a modification of the sagittal curvatures, which manifests, in most cases, in a flat back with proximal lumbar hypolordosis, thoracic hypokyphosis, and cervical hypolordosis or kyphosis [4–6].

Nevertheless, most patients with "unfused" AIS remain balanced on the sagittal plane thanks to the spine's flexibility, which allows for spontaneous equilibration [7,8].

Current correction techniques using high-density anchors allow for a relevant reduction in the coronal deformity (from 65 to 80%) [8]. In addition to coronal outcomes, sagittal results strongly affect long-term quality of life [9–11] and the degeneration of uninstrumented levels for both the cervical [12–15] and lumbar [16].

The majority of AIS procedures include thoracic spine fixation, either for the main curve (Lenke 1–4) or for the thoracic counter-curve of Lenke 6 [8,17]. Consequently, the deformity correction requires an appropriate instrumented thoracic spine alignment.

Moreover, many publications reporting AIS postoperative outcomes have emphasized the risk of thoracic hypokyphosis after posterior fusion [8,11,18,19]. Therefore, several authors have taken an interest in this problem, underlining the need to obtain a "normal" postoperative thoracic kyphosis (TK) [20–22]. The normal TK is currently accepted to be between 10° and 40° (according to Lenke's classification) or between 20° and 50° [22–24]. However, recent works have suggested that there should not be the same normal TK for all individuals but rather a patient-specific TK adapted to the individual lumbo-pelvic parameters [24–26]. Therefore, the targeted TK for each patient remains debatable, as well as its distribution (i.e., the number of vertebrae in TK) and the location of the TK apex (TKA) [22,25]. In addition, the way of measuring TK is not unanimous, with various methods being used, based on either predefined anatomical landmarks (e.g., T4–T12) or functional ones (e.g., global TK) 2,20,22].

Moreover, the insufficient restoration of TK increases the risk of proximal junctional kyphosis (PJK) or proximal junctional failure [27,28]. Indeed, PJK allows for the patient to regain their sagittal balance by accentuating the kyphosis above the fusion [26,29]. These iatrogenic PJKs come up frequently in the literature, involving up to 46% of patients, and can usually be detected early (within 4 months postoperative) [13,28]. Even if few of them require revision surgery, they can be a source of morphological disorders, pain, and long-term adjacent degeneration [28,30].

The search for a good sagittal balance after AIS surgery therefore leads to a reflection on the target values of sagittal curvatures, on their planning, and on the intraoperative execution [31–33].

The most common way to bend rods is manually, without a measured target, based on the aim and experience of the surgeon [34,35]. The use of patient-specific rods (PSR) is undoubtedly a possible response to improve sagittal balance restoration and to obtain post-operative sagittal angles that are closer to the planned ones [36–38]. This method was first utilized for adults, then, more recently, for adolescents [31,39].

This review aims to provide an update about patient-specific planning and rods in AIS, looking at the current literature.

The following topics in the publications will be analyzed:
- TK planning method;
- Manufacturing: various ways to obtain PSR;
- Comparison between programmed and achieved TK;
- PJK incidence.

2. Materials and Methods

This is a systematic review of the patient-specific planning and rods for AIS surgical correction. It has been submitted and registered to the PROSPERO website https://www.crd.york.ac.uk/PROSPERO/ (accessed on 11 January 2024) with number 414039. This report was prepared according to Preferred Reporting Items for Systematic Reviews and Meta-Analyses (PRISMA) guideline 5, as suggested by the Enhancing the QUAlity and Transparency Of health Research (EQUATOR) network (Supplemental File S1) [40].

As a literature review, ethics committee approval was not required.

Electronic databases of EMBASE, MEDLINE/PubMed, Science Direct, Scopus, and Web of Knowledge were searched from 2013 (first use of PSR) through 30 November 2023 (search date), with the following keywords: "adolescent" or "children" + "scoliosis" + "patient-specific" or "patient" and "specific", including but not limited to reports in English, French, Italian, Spanish, and Portuguese languages. We also searched Google and Google scholar to bring out the gray literature, and further reviewed them for credibility after the initial search. The literature was further checked on 4 January 2024 lest miss a more recent paper.

For the systematic review, we aimed to analyze all case series and case reports of PSR and/or patient-specific planning for AIS, including journal articles and meeting proceedings. No minimum follow-up was defined for inclusion.

Articles were further screened for interventions and were included if they clearly reported the type of treatment and the radiologic sagittal outcomes at the last follow-up.

To be comprehensive, bibliographies of relevant reviews and selected studies were examined. Reviews, historical articles, and other related documents were manually added.

Study selection was performed in two stages by paired reviewers (first and last author), screening independently and in duplicate. Titles and abstracts were screened in the first stage, followed by full-text readings of potentially eligible citations.

The same-paired reviewers extracted the data independently and in duplicate using electronic data extraction forms. Disagreements were resolved by consensus or through discussion with a third investigator (second author). The selection of the articles is summarized in the PRISMA diagram (Figure 1).

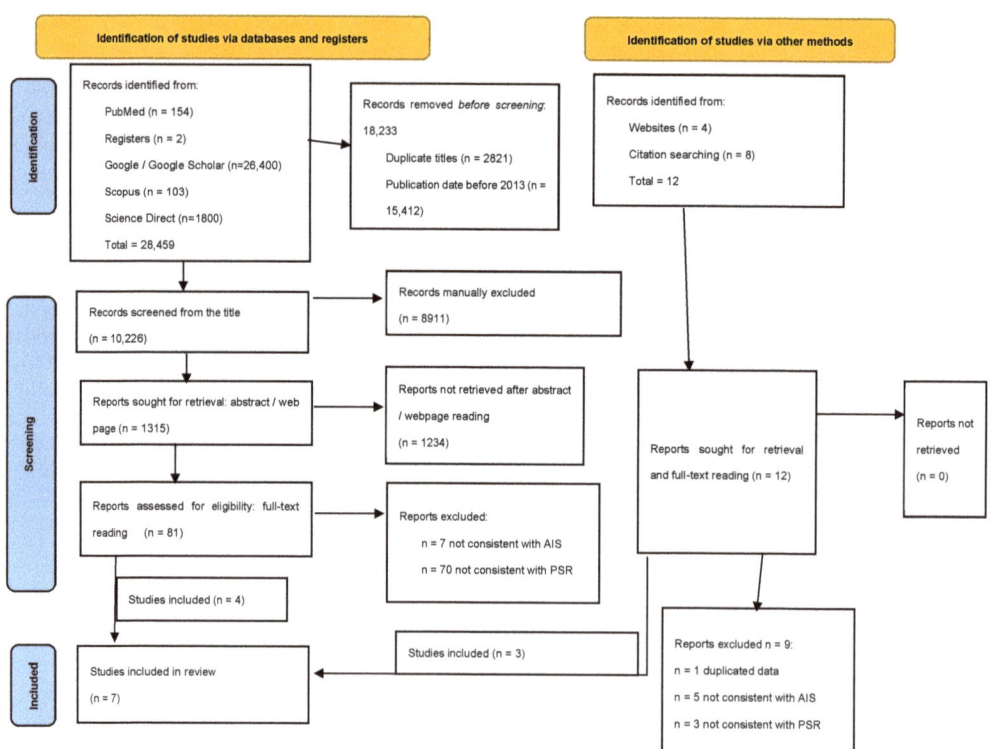

Figure 1. PRISMA flowchart.

The potential bias was assessed using the MINORS score, which evaluates non-randomized comparative studies with 12 questions and non-comparative studies with 8 questions, scoring them from 0 to 2 [41]. The sum of the points was used to grade the quality of each study: poor (<8 for non-comparative or <12 for comparative), good (9–12 for non-comparative or 13–18 for comparative), or excellent (>13 for non-comparative or >18 for comparative).

3. Results

3.1. Literature Search Results

Eight case studies of PSR and AIS were identified, exclusively from France (n = 5) or the United States (n = 3). One presented redundant data and deserved exclusion. Thus, seven studies were retained for the present analysis: four journal articles and three proceedings from international congresses, reporting on 355 patients in total [39,42–47]. An overview is provided in Table 1. The study design was mostly a cohort study (evidence level: 4), except for one comparative study versus standard rods (evidence level: 3) [48]. Six were monocentric and one was multicentric. The minimum follow-up was between 4 and 24 months.

The average MINORS score was 11.7 ± 2.2 (min. 9, max 15), resulting in good quality for six studies and excellent quality for one study (Table 1).

Table 1. Quality assessment.

General Informations				MINORS Sub-Score								
Main Author	Type of Study*	Minimum Follow-Up (Months)	Type of Paper**	A Clearly Stated Aim	Inclusion of Consecutive Patients	Prospective Collection of Data	Appropriate Endpoints	Unbiased Assessment of the Endpoint	Follow-Up Period	Loss to Follow Up <5%	Adequate Statistical Analyses	Total	Out of	Quality
Thomas	1	24	A	2	2	1	2	0	2	1	2	12	16	Good
Marya	1	6	A	2	2	1	2	1	1	0	2	11	16	Good
Solla (OTSR)	1	12	A	2	2	2	2	1	1	1	2	13	16	Excellent
Solla (ESJ)	2	12	P	2	0	1	2	1	1	0	2	9	16	Good
Alijanipour	1	12	P	2	2	1	2	0	1	0	2	15***	24	Good
Grobost/Abelin	1	6	P	1	2	2	2	1	1	0	1	10	16	Good
Ferrero	1	4	A	2	2	2	2	2	0	0	2	12	16	Good
Average		10.86		1.86	1.71	1.43	2.00	0.86	1.00	0.29	1.86	11.17	16	
Modal value	1	12	A	2	2	1	2	1	1	0	2	12		Good

* 1 = monocentric, 2 = multicentric. ** A = Article, P = Proceeding. *** 10 points from listed items + 5 points for comparative study with adequate control group with same baseline characteristics.

3.2. Radiological Planning and Analysis

Each author deliberately chose their target TK based on their experience, within ranges of 25–45°, with the highest values for the highest PI, but there was not a clear method of calculation [42–47]. The analyzed studies did not clearly report on TKA planning and the achieved position, nor on the number of vertebrae of TK and the transition points. The limits of TK measurements were T4-T12, T5-T12, global, i.e., maximum TK, or "instrumented" TK, i.e., kyphosis of the instrumented thoracic spine patients [42–47].

The programs used were mainly Surgimap® and Unid Hub® [49,50] (Table 2).

Table 2. Alignment planning programs.

Program	Online/Download?	Free/Suscription	Owner	Link to Spine Companies	Planning Author	Pros	Cons
Surgimap	Download	Basic version is free	Independent	Stryker, Globus, various	Surgeon	Free version	
Keops	Online	Subscription (but usually free for SMAIO clients)	Smaio	Smaio	SMAIO Company	Possible data sharing for scientifc studies; Radiological analysis by a third part	
Unid hub	Online	Free for Medtronic clients	Medtronic	Medtronic only	Surgeon and/or Medtronic team	Radiological analysis by a third part	Hard password; only for medtronic planning
SpineEOS	Online	Subscription	Alphatec	None	Surgeon	Link to EOS imaging	Need for EOS imaging

3.3. How to Obtain PSR

The analyzed literature showed that various strategies are currently available to obtain PSR, with each PSR company proposing its own spine fixation system (Table 3).

Table 3. Companies involved in PSR and/or pre-bent rods.

Company (Country)	Type of Technology	Type of Rods	Rod–Screw Connection	Fixation Implants
Medicrea (Fr)/Medtronic (US)	Planning and manufacture	Ti or CoCr, 6 or 5.5 or 3.5 mm, round or derotation rod with baseball-field section (2 plate faces and 2/3 of circus)	-Top connection (tulip screws)	Polyaxial, monoaxial or uniplanar pedicle screws;
			-Side connection (dome screws) with polyaxial/derotation/realignment connectors	Hooks, claws, sublaminar bands
SMAIO (Fr)	Planning and manufacture	Ti 6 or 5.5 mm, round section	Side connection	Monoaxial; screws, hooks and claws.
Nuvasive (US)	Planning and measured bending with a connected bender	Ti or CrCo, 6 or 5 mm, round section	Top connection	Polyaxial or monoaxial; screws, hooks, sublaminar bands
Robert Reid (Japan)	Manufacturing of pre-bent rods	CrCo 5.5, round section	Side connection	Polyaxial screws

Fr: France; Ti: Titanium; CrCo: Chromium–Cobalt.

The most basic way to implant rods that are similar to the planned rods should be to contour them with a manual bender according to pre-operative planning. However, this process is potentially imprecise and few articles reported on it [34,51].

A slightly more precise option to obtain quasi-PSR is to choose "best match" rods from a set of pre-bent rods of various curves and lengths (Robert-Reid Inc., Tokyo, Japan) according to preoperative planning [52]. Sudo et al. did not report rod-cutting or additional bending [53,54]. However, if required, such modifications are possible in order to fit the length of the instrumented spine and the targeted alignment. This process should be more precise than manual bending since the rods' curve is industrially measured, but the plan would probably match some approximation of the shape of pre-bent rods. Moreover, the plan would be more expensive than manual bending but there would be no notches, other than in cases of additional manual bending. Data from the literature about this process showed good sagittal results but did not address the relationship between the planning and the achieved sagittal alignment [52–54]. In a comparative study, patients with notch-free pre-bent rods had a significantly higher postoperative TK than patients with conventional, manually bent notched rods (30 vs. 24°). The rod deformation angles were significantly lower in the notch-free rods than in the notched rods on the concave side (7 vs. 13°) [52]. These results suggest that the notch-free rod can better maintain its curvature, leading to the better correction or maintenance of TK than the notched rod. To the best of our knowledge, this type of implant is only available in Japan [55].

A third option to obtain patient-specific contouring is to print a paper template in 1:1 dimensions using the digitally planned rod [42,43]. This can then be used in the operating room in a sterile envelope, allowing for the surgeon to bend the rods accordingly. Two articles are available on this process, showing a post-operative TK within +/− 5.5° of the predicted value from Marya and no significant difference for Ferrero [42,43]. Marya also reported an average under-bending of rods of < 1°. Ferrero reported good correspondence between planned and achieved lordosis (57~58°), with constructs reaching L2, L3, or L4, but different TL inflection points of about two levels between planned and implanted rods [42,43]. This process of obtaining PSR presents no additional cost compared with standard rods; however, it requires more time during surgery than pre-bent rods, and notching will be present.

Another available option to obtain the measured rod contouring during the surgery is to use a calibrated bender linked to a planning program (Bendini, Nuvasive®, San Diego, CA, USA) [56]. This process is probably precise, and is somewhat expensive due to the connected bender, but is potentially less precise and less expensive than factory-bent rods. However, notches will be present and there are currently no available results on this system's use in AIS surgery.

Finally, the most sophisticated and, probably, most precise system is the industrial manufacturing of pre-bent rods according to planning. The first company to develop this process was Medicrea, a French company of spine implants including side-connected polyaxial dome screws. Five reports are available on this [39,44–47]. In 2021, Medtronic, an international company of medical technologies including spine implants, acquired Medicrea, and currently proposes PSR's use for the side-connection Medicrea system (PASS LP®) and for the Medtronic top-connection tulip screw and hook systems (Solera®) (Table 3) [50]. In 2021, SMAIO, another French company of spine implants and programs, developed its own PSR manufacturing system, with side-connected monoaxial dome screws [57]. For these implants, there are currently no available results. This process should be the simplest for the surgeon and is probably the most precise, with no notching on the rods; however, it is quite expensive, since it requires specific manufacturing for each patient (as per "haute couture" clothing).

3.4. Radiological Outcomes

From the analyzed studies, coronal correction was between 64% and 75% [8,42].

The rate of patients with postoperative normokyphosis was between 95% and 100% [42–47] (Table 4). Solla et al. reported that factors associated with achieved TK at the last follow-up included the concave rod contouring angle and the pre-operative TK angle ($p < 0.05$) [46]. The mean difference between the pre-operative TK and the TK at last follow-up was between $-1°$ for the Cantilever technique [43] and 14° for postero-medial translation [46]. In hypokyphotic patients, the mean difference between the pre-operative and the last follow-up TK was between 14° for Cantilever technique and 20° for PMT [43,46].

Table 4. Overview of the analyzed studies.

Main Author	Year	Planning Software	Rods Material and Technology	Pre-Bent or Manually Bent	Surgical Technique and Construct	Number of Patients	Coronal Cobb Angle	TK Increase	TK Increase in Hypo-TK	Planned TK	Planned-Achieved TK	% Patients with Normal TK at Last Follow-Up	Postoperative TL Angle
Thomas [44]	2022	Unid hub	6 mm Ti, identical, Unid	Pre-bent	ST2R with Ponte osteotomies, apical sublaminar bands (n = 4)	48	63	6.4	19	30 to 40°	−3°		8° lordosis
Marya [43]	2023	Surgimap	5.5 mm Ti, asymmetrical (+20° on concave side), manually bent according to a paper template; rail on concave side, round on convex	Manually bent	Cantilever, multiple pedicle screws construct	61	68	−1	14		5° ± 4		
Solla [46]	2018	Surgimap	6 mm CoCr, asymmetrical, diamond section, Unid (+10° for concave side rod)	Pre-bent	ST2R, multiple pedicle screws construct, concave derotation	37	53	14	20	34	0°: −4 in normoK, +5 in hypo K	97% (1 patient with TK = 56°)	
Solla [47]	2020	Surgimap or Unid Hub	Unid, various: 5.5 or 6 mm, Ti or CoCr	Pre-bent	ST2R, multiple pedicle screws construct ± concave de-rotation or sublaminar bands	85	-	12	19		1°: −4 in normoK, +6 in hypo K	96% (2 patients with TK between 10 and 20°)	
Alijanipour [39]	2017	Surgimap	Mostly 6 mm Ti, identical, Unid vs. conventional "unplanned" rods	Pre-bent	ST2R with multiple pedicle screws construct	28 vs. 28	57	−2 vs. −3					significantly lordotic in C group (−7.3.) compared to PS group (−0.3, p\0.001).
Grobost/Abelin [45]	2019	Keops	5.5 mm CoCr or 6 mm Ti, identical, Unid	Pre-bent	ST2R with multiple pedicle screws construct + sublaminar bands at the apex	49	54 ± 10	10		30 ± 8	0	95%	significantly improved after surgery

Table 4. *Cont.*

Main Author	Year	Planning Software	Rods Material and Technology	Pre-Bent or Manually Bent	Surgical Technique and Construct	Number of Patients	Coronal Cobb Angle	TK Increase	TK Increase in Hypo-TK	Planned TK	Planned–Achieved TK	% Patients with Normal TK at Last Follow-Up	Postoperative TL Angle
Ferrero/Ilharreborde 2018 [42]		SpineEOS	5.5 mm CoCr identical manually bent according to a paper template	Manually bent	Translation on 1 rod; lumbar pedicle screws and thoracic sublaminar bands	47	59 ± 13	9		38	1	100%	
Sum						355							
Average	2020		5.8			51	59	7	18	34	0.67	97	
Modal value		Surgimap		Pre-bent	ST2R								

ST2R: simultaneous translation on two rods; TK: thoracic kyphosis.

Three studies reported no significant difference between the planned and achieved TK using sublaminar bands at the apex of the thoracic curves [42,44,45]. The behavior of hooks or claws at the apex of the main curve is not described with PSR. However, their use at the cranial part of the thoracic construct is reported in four studies [42,44,46,48].

The mean gap between planned and achieved TK was −3° for Thomas with 6 mm Ti rods, 0° for Solla ($p = 0.85$) with 6 mm CrCo rods, and Abelin with 5.5 CrCo or 6 mm Ti rods, 1° for Ferrero ($p = 0.98$) with 5.5 mm CrCo rods, and 5° for Marya ($p = 0.4$) with 5.5 mm Ti rods [42–48]. These data moderately suggest that using stiffer rods increases the correspondence between the PSR contour and the achieved TK.

Concerning the rods' behavior, Thomas et al., using sublaminar bands and 6 mm Ti symmetrical PSR, reported a minimal change (<1 mm), even in the hypokyphotic group, in rod deflection at 2-year follow-up, compared to the predicted rod deflection [44]. From Alijanipour et al., both maximal deflection distance (23 vs. 17 mm) and the angles of tangents to rod endpoints (30 vs. 17°) were higher for PSR than for conventional rods [39]. Solla et al. reported a visual flattening of the concave rod but did not report specific measurements and suggested the concave rods were over-contoured by 10° in cases of pre-operative hypokyphosis [46]. Concerning subgroup analysis, from over-bent 6 mm CrCo concave side rods, the mean TK gain was 20° for an expected gain of 25° in the subgroup with pre-operative hypokyphosis (<20°). Of the 17 patients in this subgroup, 10 were under-corrected (achieved TK 5° lower than expected TK) but all achieved TK > 20°. However, in the subgroup with normal preoperative kyphosis (n = 18), the mean TK gain was 8° for an expected gain of 4°. In this subgroup, 11 out of 18 were overcorrected (achieved TK was 5° higher than expected TK) [46].

In a study with 5.5 Ti rods and multiple screws, there was a significant post-operative change in TK in both the hypo- and hyper-kyphotic patient groups, resulting in patients achieving a mean TK within the 'normal' parameters of 20–40°, whereas the normokyphotic patients had a marginal, non-relevant increase in TK post-operatively [43].

The thoraco–lumbar junction was specifically analyzed in three studies: two of them obtained a straight TL junction after PSR surgery, whereas Thomas found an average of 8° of lordosis at the last follow-up, very close to the pre-operative value (7°) [43,44,47]. They also found that the sagittal TL inflection point in hypokyphotic patients shifted inferiorly, from the T9 superior endplate preoperatively to the T10 superior endplate postoperatively, which was maintained throughout the 24-month follow-up. However, the planned position of TKA was not declared.

Concerning lumbo-pelvic parameters, Ferrero reported that 21% of the patients had not achieved LL within reference values: four had hypolordosis and six had hyperlordosis [42]. Nevertheless, in 25% (n = 12), the 3D planning tool overestimated lumbar lordosis by 10° or more. Postoperative SVA was superior by 20 mm in nine cases (19%) and the C7 plumb line was anterior to the sacrum in 33% of cases (n = 16). Nevertheless, the postoperative values of TK, pelvic tilt, and SVA were not different from the planned values. Thomas also reported an LL increase, which was mainly observed in L1–L4, with no significant change in L4–S1. The pelvic parameters remained relatively unchanged. These authors observed a pelvic retroversion (PT increase and SS decrease) at 6 months, which returned to baseline at 12 or 24 months post operation. Thomas et al. found a compensatory median gain of 7° in LL by the 2-year follow-up, reaching "normal" parameters as proposed by Mac-Thiong et al. [44,58].

According to the available data, there is no PJK after PSR implantation.

4. Discussion

All authors reported high correspondence between planned and achieved TK, despite the use of different surgical techniques and rod properties.

Concerning the planned TK, the previous literature [59,60] suggested that achieving ≥23° or ≥26° of TK decreased the risk of sagittal plane decompensation and cervical malalignment following thoracic fusions for AIS. However, the best target TK for each patient was rarely explored. It seems difficult to deduce the "ideal" sagittal alignment of the spine from the deformed spine sagittal alignment, and only the pelvic parameters can provide proper orientation [3]. Abelin-Genevois et al. found that the restoration of lumbo-pelvic alignment helped to limit early degenerative changes in the free motion segments after AIS surgery [61]. This systematic review has also confirmed that the pelvic parameters are not modified by surgery at follow-up, despite some transient post-operative changes [62]. It is therefore possible to predict the best spinopelvic alignment from pre-operative pelvic parameters, as in adult spines [63,64].

Conversely, both cervical and lumbar lordosis are negatively affected by pathological thoracic kyphosis [62,65]. Postoperative TK increases have been shown to achieve a reciprocal increase in LL that has beneficial effects for a patient's future, related to the natural loss of LL with aging and disc degeneration [21]. Thomas et al. found a compensatory median gain of 7° in LL, reaching "normal" parameters [44,58]. From a previous study, Clement et al. reported an LL gain that is equal to approximately 40% of TK gain, with all the gain in proximal lumbar lordosis (PLL), while distal lumbar lordosis (DLL) equivalent to SS remained unchanged from preoperative measurements [62]. Conversely, the postoperative loss of TK is strongly associated with the reciprocal loss of LL [66]. In the same way, the increase in TK entailed an improvement in cervical lordosis related to the increase in distal cervical lordosis, with 60% of the TK increase transferred to the gain in distal cervical lordosis [65].

It has been geometrically demonstrated that global LL and GTK are dependent on pelvic parameters. The formula GTK = $2 \times$(PT+LL-PI) has been validated in adolescents and young adults without spine pathology [24,25]. Therefore, each individual has a specific TK according to their lumbo-pelvic parameters. At present, it seems necessary not to choose a given target angle for all patients (e.g., 30°), but rather to seek the correct sagittal alignment by providing the patient's "best" GTK. The calculation of the targeted GTK requires anticipating the post-operative variations in LL due to the increase in TK [62]. Then, it is easy to calculate the value of the instrumented TK from a targeted GTK.

The analyzed studies correspond to the beginning of PSR use, when the formula GTK = $2 \times$(PT-LL-PI) was unknown. Each author deliberately chose a target TK based on their experience, within ranges of 25–45°, with the highest values for the highest PI, but there was not a clear method of calculation [42–45].

When planning for LL, a similar process is available. LL can be divided into PLL and DLL [62]. PLL is calculated using the formula PT+LL-PI, considering the increase in LL linked to the increase in TK.

The length of the TK and the position of the apex should also be planned. A TKA position between T5 and T8 is frequent in the normal population. A recent study suggests apex on T8 for mild PI and T9 for high PI (type 3 or 4 of Roussouly) [25]. Other authors suggest apex on T7 or T9 [58,67]. However, the ideal TKA position for each subject is still unknown, and depends on the length of GTK between its two points of inflection, and on the harmony of the kyphosis. If the kyphosis is regular, PTK is similar to DTK, and the apex is in the middle of GTK. On the other hand, if the kyphosis is not regular, PTK and DTK are not equal, and the apex is shifted up or down. Unfortunately, the analyzed studies did not clearly report on TKA planning and the achieved position, nor did they report on the number of vertebrae of TK and the transition points. We recommend a more complete and specific assessment of sagittal results with an evaluation of the type of Roussouly, the apex of the sagittal curves, and the points of inflection.

Various options are currently available to plan sagittal correction and to implant rods corresponding to planning, ranging from the simplest and cheapest (printed rod model and manual bending) to the most expensive and precise (industrial manufacturing).

To improve the planning process, simulation tools allow for a clear definition of a targeted alignment for each patient (Table 2) [57,68,69]. Based on the literature, they seem useful for planning sagittal correction and anticipating the postoperative behavior of the corrected spine, regardless of whether the spine surgeon uses PSR [70]. Various programs are available for this purpose, with each having pros and cons: some are "independent", whereas others are linked to a specific company producing implants. Based on the principle of balance between the pelvis, LL, and TK, it is possible to simulate the GTK correction conforming to a balanced sagittal alignment.

TK planning requires a clear definition of the measurement limits, which vary across the literature, e.g., T4–T12, T5–T12, T2–T12, T1–T12, global, i.e., maximum TK, and "instrumented" TK, i.e., kyphosis of the instrumented thoracic spine patients [2,8,20,22]. This variety of measurements is somewhat confusing, even for experienced readers. From the surgical point of view, the most objective and reliable parameter is probably the "instrumented" TK, i.e., the TK of the instrumented thoracic spine, which strictly reflects the adherence (or lack of) between the planned instrumented TK and the TK achieved for the instrumented zone. However, this measure is rarely reported [46]. From the functional point of view, the most comprehensive way to assess a patient's alignment is certainly global thoracic kyphosis (GTK), which is the spinal segment in kyphosis that intervenes in the sagittal balance and is measured from the cervico-thoracic inflection point to the thoraco-lumbar inflection point [8,22,24]. GTK is characterized as having the most cranial and most caudal vertebrae, and by the position of the thoracic kyphosis apex (TKA). The horizontal line through the TKA separates GTK into proximal TK (PTK) and distal TK (DTK). However, after fusion, GTK may include both instrumented and uninstrumented thoracic segments, unless the construct covers the entire thoracic spine. Furthermore, in the case of PJK, GTK includes both instrumented TK and PJK. This concept highlights the need to measure proximal junctional angle (PJA, i.e., the sagittal angle between the proximal endplate of the upper instrumented vertebra and the superior endplate of the two supra-adjacent vertebrae above it) when assessing post-operative sagittal outcomes [26,28].

It must be pointed out that patient-specific planning requires more time than a lack of planning, for the PSR company and/or for the surgeon, but various articles and common sense suggest that planned surgery provides better outcomes than unplanned surgery [71,72]. Additionally, the planning should be prepared before the surgical procedure, allowing for the surgeon to concentrate on planning when outside the operating room and on the patient once inside [73,74].

Concerning surgical use, PSR can be implanted and connected to spine anchors like normal rods. However, the surgical strategies, the release technique (facet resection, osteotomies), the baseline characteristics, and a surgeon's skills and experience could influence the relationship between the shape of the rod and the achieved sagittal alignment [75–77].

Monoaxial screws, if implanted parallel to the superior plateau, should pull each vertebra perpendicular to the rod and achieve a good spine adherence to rod shape; however, this comes at the cost of bending stress, and is potentially detrimental to the stability of the screws [78]. Contrarily, monoaxial screws with a "quirky" direction not parallel to the endplate should increase the work required to connect them to the rod and entail a less precise adherence to the planned alignment. These statements are less absolute for polyaxial screws, which tolerate a certain amount of obliquity and are less constraining but should result in a less precise congruence with the planned alignment [79]. However, there are currently no reports on PSR and monoaxial screws.

Moreover, the type of connection between screws and rods (top-loading vs. lateral connection) may influence the relationship between the shape of the rod and the achieved sagittal alignment, with side-connections probably providing better congruence in the case of severe sagittal disorder [80].

Three studies reported encouraging outcomes regarding the use of sublaminar bands at the apex of thoracic curves. Thomas et al. postulated that the use of sublaminar double bands in the area of apical hypokyphosis associated with postero-medial translation (PMT) resulted in a minimal change in rod shape. Similarly, both Grobost and Ferrero reported no difference between the simulated model and the postoperative sagittal parameters [42,44,45].

In hypokyphotic patients, the mean difference between pre-operative TK and TK at last follow-up was higher with the translation technique than for the cantilever. It is worth noting that both the minimum and maximum values of the difference between expected and achieved TK concerned screw-based constructs, suggesting that the type of vertebral implants is less relevant than the aim of the surgeon and the correction technique [43,46]. In the previous literature, the correction technique seems to play an important role. A recent multicenter study on 562 AIS showed that in situ bending and cantilever resulted in a postoperative decrease in TK of about 5°, whereas rod rotation and PMT resulted in an increase in TK (of +7° and +16°, respectively) [8]. It therefore seems better to use a reduction technique capable of reaching a target TK, especially in the case of hypokyphosis. Moreover, six out of seven studies from the present review concern the PMT technique, which seems more effective in adapting the spine to the plan and not the plan to the existing sagittal disorder [41,43–47]. On the other hand, in situ bending should not be used as the main correction technique with PSR because it implies per-operative rod contouring. However, a certain amount of in situ bending could be added after PMT or rod rotation to increase coronal correction, but this potentially decreases sagittal correction [8]. Conversely, if the surgeon wants to continue using their preferred cantilever technique, we would suggest over-bent rods, especially in cases of hypokyphosis [8].

Rod-flattening was frequently observed due to a compromise between the stiffness of the spine and the corrective power of the construct, especially in severe pre-operative hypokyphosis [46]. This can be anticipated, at least for moderate AIS and reproducible surgical techniques. With conventional rods, Cidambi et al. reported rod-flattening with a decrease in deflection of 13 mm and a 21° decrease in rod angle with 5.5 mm stainless steel rods [81]. Abe et al. reported a rod-flattening of 16° in patients treated with 6 mm Ti rods [82]. Kluck et al. reported that concave rods flattened, on average, by ~20°, whereas the average convex rod angle increased by 4° [83]. Sia et al. reported that the curvature of the titanium rod and cobalt chrome rod decreased from 60° to 37°, and 51° to 28°, respectively [84]. Le Naveaux and Gay recommended over-contouring the concave rod by 13° to induce an increase in postoperative TK and apical derotation [85,86].

In the available data, there is no PJK after PSR implantation. Even if this complication is underreported, it has been specifically assessed in three studies [41–43], whereas the common rate from the literature is between 7% and 46% [13,28–30]. Despite the multifactorial etiology, a good sagittal alignment is confirmed to be a strong protective factor [29,87]. The use of hooks or claws at the proximal part of the thoracic construct could have played a role in the absence of PJK, as previously reported with standard rods [88–90].

5. Limitations

The limits of the current review include the small number of subjects in the published studies. Moreover, most papers suffer from industry support, a moderate level of evidence (3 or 4), the short and different lengths of the observation periods, a moderate risk of bias with only one comparative study, and the limited amount of available data. Furthermore, the TK measurements are not the same for all studies.

6. Future Directions

The next steps should include multicenter studies using various surgical and manufacturing strategies to assess:

- How the properties of the rod (diameter, section, material, notched vs. not notched), surgical factors (type and density of implants, type of rod–screw connection, correction and release technique), and baseline variates (spine stiffness, pre-operative TK, patient-related factors, etc.) might influence the relationship between the plan and the achieved alignment;
- If the achieved plan, including the regularity of TK, the position of the apex, and the transition points between TK and adjacent curves, was optimal concerning the postoperative modifications to global alignment, adjacent sagittal curves, and quality

of life. For this, TK planning requires a clear definition of the measurement limits, apex, and the number of vertebrae included.

To fine-tune planning, sagittal results should be predictable at both instrumented and uninstrumented levels. If the latter are known from the literature, the former should be analyzed for each surgeon, depending on the implants, the correction technique, and human factors.

Further clinical evaluations are underway to confirm the benefits of planning sagittal results and implanting PSRs that are strictly bent following the planning, allowing for a quantifiable and reproducible sagittal correction.

7. Conclusions

Various options are currently available to plan sagittal corrections and to implant rods corresponding to planning.

The outcomes of the first PSR experiences in AIS surgery are encouraging, showing a good correspondence between the expected TK and the achieved TK, and the absence of PJK.

Current data suggest using stiff, over-bent, concave side rods, and translation techniques for correction, in cases of preoperative hypokyphosis.

Supplementary Materials: The following supporting information can be downloaded at: https://www.mdpi.com/article/10.3390/children11010106/s1, Supplemental File S1: PRISMA checklist.

Author Contributions: Conceptualization, F.S., J.-L.C. and B.I.; methodology, F.S.; validation, F.S., E.O.R., C.M.B., M.M. and E.O.R.; formal analysis, F.S. and C.M.B.; investigation, F.S. and M.M.; data curation, F.S. and J.-L.C.; writing—original draft preparation, F.S., V.R., M.M. and E.O.R.; writing—review and editing, B.I., J.-L.C., M.M., C.M.B., V.R. and E.O.R.; All authors have read and agreed to the published version of the manuscript.

Funding: Article Processing Charges were provided by: SMAIO (Saint-Priest, Fr) and Lenval Foundation (Nice, Fr).

Institutional Review Board Statement: Ethical review and approval were waived for this study due to its nature (systematic review).

Informed Consent Statement: Not applicable.

Data Availability Statement: All data are included in the article or in the tables.

Acknowledgments: One of the authors (FS) performed this study in the framework of the International PhD in Innovation Sciences and Technologies of the University of Cagliari.

Conflicts of Interest: FS received support for congresses from Medtronic and Euros; BI is a consultant for Zimmer Biomet, Medtronic and Implanet; JLC receives royalties from Medtronic unrelated to this study; the other authors declare no conflicts of interest.

References

1. Mak, T.; Cheung, P.W.H.; Zhang, T.; Cheung, J.P.Y. Patterns of coronal and sagittal deformities in adolescent idiopathic scoliosis. *BMC Musculoskelet. Disord.* **2021**, *22*, 44. [CrossRef]
2. Gardner, A.; Berryman, F.; Pynsent, P. The kyphosis–lordosis difference parameter and its utility in understanding the pathogenesis of adolescent idiopathic scoliosis. *BMC Res. Notes* **2022**, *15*, 178. [CrossRef] [PubMed]
3. Post, M.; Verdun, S.; Roussouly, P.; Abelin-Genevois, K. New sagittal classification of AIS: Validation by 3D characterization. *Eur. Spine J.* **2019**, *28*, 551–558. [CrossRef] [PubMed]
4. Fruergaard, S.; Jain, M.J.; Deveza, L.; Liu, D.; Heydemann, J.; Ohrt-Nissen, S.; Dragsted, C.; Gehrchen, M.; Dahl, B.; Texas Children's Hospital Spine Study Group. Evaluation of a new sagittal classification system in adolescent idiopathic scoliosis. *Eur. Spine J.* **2020**, *29*, 744–753. [CrossRef] [PubMed]
5. Ritzman, T.F.; Floccari, L.V. The Sagittal Plane in Spinal Fusion for Adolescent Idiopathic Scoliosis. *J. Am. Acad. Orthop. Surg.* **2022**, *30*, e957–e967. [CrossRef] [PubMed]
6. Zhang, C.M.; Wang, Y.; Yu, J.; Jin, F.; Zhang, Y.; Zhao, Y.; Fu, Y.; Zhang, K.; Wang, J.; Dai, L.; et al. Analysis of sagittal curvature and its influencing factors in adolescent idiopathic scoliosis. *Medicine* **2021**, *100*, e26274. [CrossRef]

7. Iimura, T.; Ueda, H.; Inami, S.; Moridaira, H.; Takeuchi, D.; Aoki, H.; Taneichi, H. Thoracic kyphosis in light of lumbosacral alignment in thoracic adolescent idiopathic scoliosis: Recognition of thoracic hypokyphosis and therapeutic implications. *BMC Musculoskelet. Disord.* **2022**, *23*, 414. [CrossRef]
8. Pesenti, S.; Clément, J.-L.; Ilharreborde, B.; Morin, C.; Charles, Y.P.; Parent, H.F.; Violas, P.; Szadkowski, M.; Boissière, L.; Jouve, J.-L.; et al. Comparison of four correction techniques for posterior spinal fusion in adolescent idiopathic scoliosis. *Eur. Spine J.* **2022**, *31*, 1028–1035. [CrossRef]
9. Boeckenfoerde, K.; Boevingloh, A.S.; Gosheger, G.; Bockholt, S.; Lampe, L.P.; Lange, T. Risk Factors of Proximal Junctional Kyphosis in Adolescent Idiopathic Scoliosis—The Spinous Processes and Proximal Rod Contouring. *J. Clin. Med.* **2022**, *11*, 6098. [CrossRef]
10. Pasha, S.; Ilharreborde, B.; Baldwin, K. Sagittal Spinopelvic Alignment After Posterior Spinal Fusion in Adolescent Idiopathic Scoliosis: A Systematic Review and Meta-analysis. *Spine* **2019**, *44*, 41–52. [CrossRef]
11. Bodendorfer, B.M.; Shah, S.A.; Bastrom, T.P.; Lonner, B.S.; Yaszay, B.; Samdani, A.F.; Miyanji, F.; Cahill, P.J.; Sponseller, P.D.; Betz, R.R.; et al. Restoration of Thoracic Kyphosis in Adolescent Idiopathic Scoliosis Over a Twenty-year Period: Are We Getting Better? *Spine* **2020**, *45*, 1625–1633. [CrossRef] [PubMed]
12. Garg, B.; Mehta, N.; Gupta, A.; Sugumar, P.A.A.; Shetty, A.P.; Basu, S.; Jakkepally, S.; Gowda, S.D.; Babu, J.N.; Chhabra, H.S. Cervical sagittal alignment in Lenke 1 adolescent idiopathic scoliosis and assessment of its alteration with surgery: A retrospective, multi-centric study. *Spine Deform.* **2021**, *9*, 1559–1568. [CrossRef]
13. Alzakri, A.; Vergari, C.; Van den Abbeele, M.; Gille, O.; Skalli, W.; Obeid, I. Global Sagittal Alignment and Proximal Junctional Kyphosis in Adolescent Idiopathic Scoliosis. *Spine Deform.* **2019**, *7*, 236–244. [CrossRef] [PubMed]
14. Lin, A.B.; Skaggs, D.L.M.; Andras, L.M.; Tolo, V.; Tamrazi, B.; Illingworth, K.D. Increasing Cervical Kyphosis Correlates With Cervical Degenerative Disc Disease in Patients With Adolescent Idiopathic Scoliosis. *Spine* **2023**. online ahead of print. [CrossRef] [PubMed]
15. Young, E.; Regan, C.; Currier, B.L.; Yaszemski, M.J.; Larson, A.N. At Mean 30-Year Follow-Up, Cervical Spine Disease Is Common and Associated with Thoracic Hypokyphosis after Pediatric Treatment of Adolescent Idiopathic Scoliosis. *J. Clin. Med.* **2022**, *11*, 6064. [CrossRef] [PubMed]
16. Bernstein, P.; Hentschel, S.; Platzek, I.; Hühne, S.; Ettrich, U.; Hartmann, A.; Seifert, J. Thoracal flat back is a risk factor for lumbar disc degeneration after scoliosis surgery. *Spine J.* **2014**, *14*, 925–932. [CrossRef] [PubMed]
17. Lenke, L.G.; Edwards, C.C.I.; Bridwell, K.H. The lenke classification of adolescent idiopathic scoliosis: How it organizes curve patterns as a template to perform selective fusions of the spine. *Spine* **2003**, *28*, S199–S207. [CrossRef]
18. Sullivan, T.B.; Bastrom, T.P.; Bartley, C.E.; Dolan, L.A.; Weinstein, S.L.; Newton, P.O. More severe thoracic idiopathic scoliosis is associated with a greater three-dimensional loss of thoracic kyphosis. *Spine Deform.* **2020**, *8*, 1205–1211. [CrossRef]
19. Schlösser, T.P.; Abelin-Genevois, K.; Homans, J.; Pasha, S.; Kruyt, M.; Roussouly, P.; Shah, S.A.; Castelein, R.M. Comparison of different strategies on three-dimensional correction of AIS: Which plane will suffer? *Eur. Spine J.* **2021**, *30*, 645–652. [CrossRef]
20. Winter, R.B.; Lonstein, J.E.; Denis, F. Sagittal spinal alignment: The true measurement, norms, and description of correction for thoracic kyphosis. *J. Spinal Disord. Tech.* **2009**, *22*, 311–314. [CrossRef]
21. Zappalá, M.; Lightbourne, S.; Heneghan, N.R. The relationship between thoracic kyphosis and age, and normative values across age groups: A systematic review of healthy adults. *J. Orthop. Surg. Res.* **2021**, *16*, 447. [CrossRef] [PubMed]
22. Laouissat, F.; Sebaaly, A.; Gehrchen, M.; Roussouly, P. Classification of normal sagittal spine alignment: Refounding the Roussouly classification. *Eur. Spine J.* **2018**, *27*, 2002–2011. [CrossRef]
23. Iyer, S.; Lenke, L.G.; Nemani, V.M.; Albert, T.J.; Sides, B.A.; Metz, L.N.; Cunningham, M.E.; Kim, H.J. Variations in Sagittal Alignment Parameters Based on Age: A Prospective Study of Asymptomatic Volunteers Using Full-Body Radiographs. *Spine* **2016**, *41*, 1826–1836. [CrossRef] [PubMed]
24. Clément, J.-L.; Solla, F.; Amorese, V.; Oborocianu, I.; Rosello, O.; Rampal, V. Lumbopelvic parameters can be used to predict thoracic kyphosis in adolescents. *Eur. Spine J.* **2020**, *29*, 2281–2286. [CrossRef] [PubMed]
25. Solla, F.; Ilharreborde, B.; Blondel, B.; Prost, S.; Bauduin, E.; Laouissat, F.; Riouallon, G.; Wolff, S.; Challier, V.; Obeid, I.; et al. Can Lumbopelvic Parameters Be Used to Predict Thoracic Kyphosis at all Ages? A National Cross-Sectional Study. *Glob. Spine J.* **2022**, 21925682221134039. [CrossRef] [PubMed]
26. Clément, J.-L.; Pesenti, S.; Ilharreborde, B.; Morin, C.; Charles, Y.-P.; Parent, H.-F.; Violas, P.; Szadkowski, M.; Boissière, L.; Solla, F. Proximal junctional kyphosis is a rebalancing spinal phenomenon due to insufficient postoperative thoracic kyphosis after adolescent idiopathic scoliosis surgery. *Eur. Spine J.* **2021**, *30*, 1988–1997. [CrossRef] [PubMed]
27. Hostin, R.A.; Yeramaneni, S.; Gum, J.L.; Smith, J.S. Clinical and Economic Impact of Proximal Junctional Kyphosis on Pediatric and Adult Spinal Deformity Patients. *Int. J. Spine Surg.* **2023**, *17*, S9–S17. [CrossRef]
28. Erkilinc, M.; Baldwin, K.D.; Pasha, S.; Mistovich, R.J. Proximal junctional kyphosis in pediatric spinal deformity surgery: A systematic review and critical analysis. *Spine Deform.* **2022**, *10*, 257–266. [CrossRef]
29. Ferrero, E.; Bocahut, N.; Lefevre, Y.; Roussouly, P.; Pesenti, S.; Lakhal, W.; Odent, T.; Morin, C.; Clement, J.-L.; Compagnon, R.; et al. Proximal junctional kyphosis in thoracic adolescent idiopathic scoliosis: Risk factors and compensatory mechanisms in a multicenter national cohort. *Eur. Spine J.* **2018**, *27*, 2241–2250. [CrossRef]
30. Cerpa, M.; Sardar, Z.; Lenke, L. Revision surgery in proximal junctional kyphosis. *Eur. Spine J.* **2020**, *29*, 78–85. [CrossRef]

31. Barton, C.; Noshchenko, A.; Patel, V.; Kleck, C.; Burger, E. Early Experience and Initial Outcomes with Patient-Specific Spine Rods for Adult Spinal Deformity. *Orthopedics* **2016**, *39*, 79–86. [CrossRef] [PubMed]
32. El Rahal, A.; Solla, F.; Fière, V.; Toquart, A.; Barrey, C.Y. *Spine Surgery. Case-Based Approach*; Sagittal balance and preoperative planning; Springer Nature: Berlin, Germany, 2019; pp. 447–458.
33. Branche, K.; Netsanet, R.; Noshchenko, A.; Burger, E.; Patel, V.; Ou-Yang, D.; Kleck, C.J. Radius of Curvature in Patient-Specific Short Rod Constructs Versus Standard Pre-Bent Rods. *Int. J. Spine Surg.* **2020**, *14*, 944–948. [CrossRef]
34. Sardi, J.P.; Ames, C.P.; Coffey, S.; Good, C.; Dahl, B.; Kraemer, P.; Gum, J.; Devito, D.; Brayda-Bruno, M.; Lee, R.; et al. Accuracy of Rod Contouring to Desired Angles with and without a Template: Implications for Achieving Desired Spinal Alignment and Outcomes. *Glob. Spine J.* **2023**, *13*, 425–431. [CrossRef] [PubMed]
35. Solla, F.; Barrey, C.Y.; Burger, E.; Kleck, C.J.; Fière, V. Patient-specific Rods for Surgical Correction of Sagittal Imbalance in Adults: Technical Aspects and Preliminary Results. *Clin. Spine Surg.* **2019**, *32*, 80–86. [CrossRef] [PubMed]
36. Prost, S.; Farah, K.; Pesenti, S.; Tropiano, P.; Fuentes, S.; Blondel, B. "Patient-specific" rods in the management of adult spinal deformity. One-year radiographic results of a prospective study about 86 patients. *Neurochirurgie* **2020**, *66*, 162–167. [CrossRef]
37. Prost, S.; Pesenti, S.; Farah, K.; Tropiano, P.; Fuentes, S.; Blondel, B. Adult Spinal Deformities: Can Patient-Specific Rods Change the Preoperative Planning into Clinical Reality? Feasibility Study and Preliminary Results about 77 Cases. *Adv. Orthop.* **2020**, *2020*, 6120580. [CrossRef] [PubMed]
38. Sadrameli, S.S.; Boghani, Z.; Iii, W.J.S.; Holman, P.J. Utility of Patient-Specific Rod Instrumentation in Deformity Correction: Single Institution Experience. *Spine Surg. Relat. Res.* **2020**, *4*, 256–260. [CrossRef]
39. Alijanipour, P.; Heffernan, M.J.; Baldwin, N.K.; King, A.G. Radiographic comparison of patient-specific (ps) and manually contoured conventional (c) rods in adolescent idiopathic scoliosis (ais) surgery. *Eur. Spine J.* **2017**, *26* (Suppl. S2), S251–S291.
40. Page, M.J.; McKenzie, J.E.; Bossuyt, P.M.; Boutron, I.; Hoffmann, T.C.; Mulrow, C.D.; Shamseer, L.; Tetzlaff, J.M.; Akl, E.A.; Brennan, S.E.; et al. The PRISMA 2020 statement: An updated guideline for reporting systematic reviews. *Int. J. Surg.* **2021**, *88*, 105906. [CrossRef]
41. Slim, K.; Nini, E.; Forestier, D.; Kwiatkowski, F.; Panis, Y.; Chipponi, J. Methodological index for non-randomized studies (MINORS): Development and validation of a new instrument. *ANZ J. Surg.* **2003**, *73*, 712–716. [CrossRef]
42. Ferrero, E.; Mazda, K.; Simon, A.-L.; Ilharreborde, B. Preliminary experience with SpineEOS, a new software for 3D planning in AIS surgery. *Eur. Spine J.* **2018**, *27*, 2165–2174. [CrossRef]
43. Marya, S.; Elmalky, M.; Schroeder, A.; Tambe, A. Correction of Thoracic Hypokyphosis in Adolescent Scoliosis Using Patient-Specific Rod Templating. *Healthcare* **2023**, *11*, 980. [CrossRef] [PubMed]
44. Thomas, E.S.; Boyer, N.; Meyers, A.; Aziz, H.; Aminian, A. Restoration of thoracic kyphosis in adolescent idiopathic scoliosis with patient-specific rods: Did the preoperative plan match postoperative sagittal alignment? *Eur. Spine J.* **2023**, *32*, 190–201. [CrossRef] [PubMed]
45. Grobost, P.; Chevillotte, T.; Verdun, S.; Abelin Genevois, K. Tiges sur Mesure pour la Correction Chirurgicale des ais- Application des Principes de la Nouvelle Classification ais Sagittale. In Proceedings of SFCR Congress, Strasbourg. 2019. Available online: https://www.sfcr.fr/uploads/media/default/0001/04/recueil-des-resumes-ok-20190709092413.pdf (accessed on 15 October 2023).
46. Solla, F.; Clément, J.-L.; Cunin, V.; Bertoncelli, C.M.; Fière, V.; Rampal, V. Patient-specific rods for thoracic kyphosis correction in adolescent idiopathic scoliosis surgery: Preliminary results. *Orthop. Traumatol. Surg. Res.* **2020**, *106*, 159–165. [CrossRef]
47. Solla, F.; Cunin, V.; Haddad, E.; Laquièvre, A.; Fière, V.; Dohin, B.; Clément, J.L. Analysis of 85 adolescent idiopathic scoliosis patients corrected with patient specific rods with a minimum of 1 year follow-up. *Eur. Spine J.* **2021**, *30*, 237–277. [CrossRef]
48. Marx, R.G.; Wilson, S.M.; Swiontkowski, M.F. Updating the Assignment of Levels of Evidence. *J. Bone Jt. Surg. Am.* **2015**, *97*, 1–2. [CrossRef]
49. Surgimap. Available online: https://www.surgimap.com/ (accessed on 5 December 2023).
50. Medtronic Unid Hub. Available online: https://platformous.medicrea.com/Account/ (accessed on 5 December 2023).
51. Langlais, T.; Bouy, A.; Eloy, G.; Mainard, N.; Skalli, W.; Vergari, C.; Vialle, R. Sagittal plane assessment of manual concave rod bending for posterior correction in adolescents with idiopathic thoracic scoliosis (Lenke 1 and 3). *Orthop. Traumatol. Surg. Res.* **2023**, *109*, 103654. [CrossRef]
52. Sudo, H.; Tachi, H.; Kokabu, T.; Yamada, K.; Iwata, A.; Endo, T.; Takahata, M.; Abe, Y.; Iwasaki, N. In vivo deformation of anatomically pre-bent rods in thoracic adolescent idiopathic scoliosis. *Sci. Rep.* **2021**, *11*, 12622. [CrossRef]
53. Tachi, H.; Kato, K.; Abe, Y.; Kokabu, T.; Yamada, K.; Iwasaki, N.; Sudo, H. Surgical Outcome Prediction Using a Four-Dimensional Planning Simulation System with Finite Element Analysis Incorporating Pre-bent Rods in Adolescent Idiopathic Scoliosis: Simulation for Spatiotemporal Anatomical Correction Technique. *Front. Bioeng. Biotechnol.* **2021**, *9*, 746902. [CrossRef]
54. Sudo, H. Four-Dimensional Anatomical Spinal Reconstruction in Thoracic Adolescent Idiopathic Scoliosis. *JBJS Essent. Surg. Tech.* **2022**, *12*, e21.00038. [CrossRef]
55. Robert Reid. Available online: https://www.robert-reid.co.jp/english/ (accessed on 21 December 2023).
56. Nuvasive. Available online: https://www.nuvasive.com/procedures/featured-offerings/bendini/ (accessed on 5 December 2023).
57. SMAIO and KEOPS. Available online: https://smaio.com/e-ifu/archives/rev_a/KROD-IMP-IFU-UE-EN_Rev_a.pdf (accessed on 5 December 2023).

58. Gutman, G.; Labelle, H.; Barchi, S.; Roussouly, P.; Berthonnaud, E.; Mac-Thiong, J.-M. Normal sagittal parameters of global spinal balance in children and adolescents: A prospective study of 646 asymptomatic subjects. *Eur. Spine J.* **2016**, *25*, 3650–3657. [CrossRef] [PubMed]
59. Rothenfluh, D.A.; Stratton, A.; Nnadi, C.; Beresford-Cleary, N. A Critical Thoracic Kyphosis Is Required to Prevent Sagittal Plane Deterioration in Selective Thoracic Fusions in Lenke I and II AIS. *Eur. Spine J.* **2019**, *28*, 3066–3075. [CrossRef] [PubMed]
60. Hwang, S.W.; Samdani, A.F.; Tantorski, M.; Cahill, P.; Nydick, J.; Fine, A.; Betz, R.R.; Antonacci, M.D. Cervical Sagittal Plane Decompensation after Surgery for Adolescent Idiopathic Scoliosis: An Effect Imparted by Postoperative Thoracic Hypokyphosis. *J. Neurosurg. Spine* **2011**, *15*, 491–496. [CrossRef] [PubMed]
61. Abelin-Genevois, K.; Estivalezes, E.; Briot, J.; Sévely, A.; De Gauzy, J.S.; Swider, P. Spino-pelvic alignment influences disc hydration properties after AIS surgery: A prospective MRI-based study. *Eur. Spine J.* **2015**, *24*, 1183–1190. [CrossRef]
62. Clément, J.-L.; Pelletier, Y.; Solla, F.; Rampal, V. Surgical increase in thoracic kyphosis increases unfused lumbar lordosis in selective fusion for thoracic adolescent idiopathic scoliosis. *Eur. Spine J.* **2019**, *28*, 581–589. [CrossRef]
63. Basu, S.; Solanki, A.; Patel, D.; Lenke, L.G.; Silva, F.E.; Biswas, A. Normal spino-pelvic parameters and correlation between lumbar lordosis (LL) and pelvic incidence (PI) in children and adolescents in Indian population. *Spine Deform.* **2021**, *9*, 941–948. [CrossRef]
64. Ignasiak, D. A novel method for prediction of postoperative global sagittal alignment based on full-body musculoskeletal modeling and posture optimization. *J. Biomech.* **2020**, *102*, 109324. [CrossRef]
65. Clement, J.-L.; Le Goff, L.; Oborocianu, I.; Rosello, O.; Bertoncelli, C.; Solla, F.; Rampal, V. Surgical increase in thoracic kyphosis predicts increase of cervical lordosis after thoracic fusion for adolescent idiopathic scoliosis. *Eur. Spine J.* **2021**, *30*, 3550–3556. [CrossRef]
66. Matsumoto, H.; Colacchio, N.D.; Schwab, F.J.; Lafage, V.; Roye, D.P.; Vitale, M.G. Flatback Revisited: Reciprocal Loss of Lumbar Lordosis Following Selective Thoracic Fusion in the Setting of Adolescent Idiopathic Scoliosis. *Spine Deform.* **2015**, *3*, 345–351. [CrossRef]
67. Sebaaly, A.; Silvestre, C.; Rizkallah, M.; Grobost, P.; Chevillotte, T.; Kharrat, K.; Roussouly, P. Revisiting thoracic kyphosis: A normative description of the thoracic sagittal curve in an asymptomatic population. *Eur. Spine J.* **2021**, *30*, 1184–1189. [CrossRef]
68. Maillot, C.; Ferrero, E.; Fort, D.; Heyberger, C.; Le Huec, J.-C. Reproducibility and repeatability of a new computerized software for sagittal spinopelvic and scoliosis curvature radiological measurements: Keops®. *Eur. Spine J.* **2015**, *24*, 1574–1581. [CrossRef]
69. SpineEOS. Available online: https://www.eos-imaging.com/us/our-expertise/advanced-orthopedic-solutions/3d-surgical-planning-tools (accessed on 5 December 2023).
70. Akbar, M.; Terran, J.; Ames, C.P.; Lafage, V.; Schwab, F. Use of surgimap spine in sagittal plane analysis, osteotomy planning, and correction calculation. *Neurosurg. Clin. N. Am.* **2013**, *24*, 163–172. [CrossRef] [PubMed]
71. Pu, J.J.M.; I Lo, A.W.; Wong, M.C.M.; Choi, W.-S.M.; Ho, G.M.; Yang, W.-F.M.; Su, Y.-X. A quantitative comparison of bone resection margin distances in virtual surgical planning versus histopathology: A prospective study. *Int. J. Surg.* **2023**. online ahead of print. [CrossRef] [PubMed]
72. Jia, S.; Weng, Y.; Wang, K.; Qi, H.; Yang, Y.; Ma, C.; Lu, W.W.; Wu, H. Performance evaluation of an AI-based preoperative planning software application for automatic selection of pedicle screws based on computed tomography images. *Front. Surg.* **2023**, *10*, 1247527. [CrossRef] [PubMed]
73. Pasha, S.; Shah, S.; Newton, P.; Group, H.S. Machine Learning Predicts the 3D Outcomes of Adolescent Idiopathic Scoliosis Surgery Using Patient–Surgeon Specific Parameters. *Spine* **2021**, *46*, 579–587. [CrossRef]
74. Bruschi, A.; Donati, D.M.; Di Bella, C. What to choose in bone tumour resections? Patient specific instrumentation versus surgical navigation: A systematic review. *J. Bone Oncol.* **2023**, *42*, 100503. [CrossRef]
75. Schlager, B.; Großkinsky, M.; Ruf, M.; Wiedenhöfer, B.; Akbar, M.; Wilke, H.-J. Range of surgical strategies for individual adolescent idiopathic scoliosis cases: Evaluation of a multi-centre survey. *Spine Deform.* **2023**, *12*, 1–12. [CrossRef]
76. Sakai, D.; Tanaka, M.; Takahashi, J.; Taniguchi, Y.; Schol, J.; Hiyama, A.; Misawa, H.; Kuraishi, S.; Oba, H.; Matsubayashi, Y.; et al. Cobalt-chromium versus titanium alloy rods for correction of adolescent idiopathic scoliosis based on 1-year follow-up: A multicenter randomized controlled clinical trial. *J. Neurosurg. Spine* **2021**, *34*, 897–906. [CrossRef]
77. Wang, F.; Chen, K.; Ji, T.; Ma, Y.; Huang, H.; Zhou, P.; Wei, X.; Chen, Z.; Bai, Y. Do hypokyphotic adolescent idiopathic scoliosis patients treated with Ponte osteotomy obtain a better clinical efficacy? A preliminary retrospective study. *J. Orthop. Surg. Res.* **2022**, *17*, 491. [CrossRef]
78. Wang, X.; Aubin, C.-E.; Crandall, D.; Labelle, H. Biomechanical comparison of force levels in spinal instrumentation using monoaxial versus multi degree of freedom postloading pedicle screws. *Spine* **2011**, *36*, E95–E104. [CrossRef]
79. Prost, S.; Pesenti, S.; Farah, K.; Tropiano, P.; Fuentes, S.; Blondel, B. Sagittal reduction of spinal deformity: Superior versus lateral screw-rod connection. *Orthop. Traumatol. Surg. Res.* **2021**, *107*, 102954. [CrossRef] [PubMed]
80. Yao, W.; Zhou, T.; Huang, K.; Dai, M.; Mo, F.; Xu, J.; Cao, Z.; Lai, Q.; Xie, B.; Guo, R.; et al. A comparison of monoaxial pedicle screw versus polyaxial pedicle screw in short-segment posterior fixation for the treatment of thoracolumbar fractured vertebra. *Ann. Transl. Med.* **2021**, *9*, 669. [CrossRef] [PubMed]
81. Cidambi, K.R.; Glaser, D.A.; Bastrom, T.P.; Nunn, T.N.; Ono, T.; Newton, P.O. Postoperative changes in spinal rod contour in adolescent idiopathic scoliosis: An in vivo deformation study. *Spine* **2012**, *37*, 1566–1572. [CrossRef] [PubMed]

82. Abe, Y.; Ito, M.; Abumi, K.; Sudo, H.; Salmingo, R.; Tadano, S. Scoliosis corrective force estimation from the implanted rod deformation using 3D-FEM analysis. *Scoliosis* **2015**, *10*, S2. [CrossRef]
83. Kluck, D.; Newton, P.O.; Sullivan, T.B.; Yaszay, B.; Jeffords, M.; Bastrom, T.P.M.; Bartley, C.E.M. A 3D Parameter Can Guide Concave Rod Contour for the Correction of Hypokyphosis in Adolescent Idiopathic Scoliosis. *Spine* **2020**, *45*, E1264–E1271. [CrossRef]
84. Sia, U.; Tan, B.; Teo, Y.; Wong, C. Post-implantation Deformation of Titanium Rod and Cobalt Chrome Rod in Adolescent Idiopathic Scoliosis. *Malays. Orthop. J.* **2019**, *13*, 14–19. [CrossRef] [PubMed]
85. Le Navéaux, F.; Aubin, C.-E.; Parent, S.; Newton, P.O.; Labelle, H. 3D rod shape changes in adolescent idiopathic scoliosis instrumentation: How much does it impact correction? *Eur. Spine J.* **2017**, *26*, 1676–1683. [CrossRef]
86. Gay, M.; Wang, X.; Ritzman, T.; Floccari, L.; Schwend, R.M.; Aubin, C.-E. Biomechanical analysis of rod contouring in posterior spinal instrumentation and fusion for 3D correction of adolescent idiopathic scoliosis. *Spine Deform.* **2023**, *11*, 1–8. [CrossRef]
87. Zhang, Z.; Zhou, Q.; Zhu, C.; Liu, L.-M.; Song, Y.-M.; Yang, X. Restoring the ideal Roussouly sagittal alignment in Lenke 5 adolescent idiopathic scoliosis patients: A method for decreasing the risk of proximal junctional kyphosis. *Eur. Spine J.* **2023**. *Online ahead of print*. [CrossRef]
88. Ogura, Y.; Glassman, S.D.; Sucato, D.; Hresko, M.T.; Carreon, L.Y. Incidence of Proximal Junctional Kyphosis with Pedicle Screws at Upper Instrumented Vertebrae in Posterior Spinal Fusion for Adolescent Idiopathic Scoliosis. *Glob. Spine J.* **2021**, *11*, 1019–1024. [CrossRef]
89. Tsirikos, A.I.; McMillan, T.E. All Pedicle Screw versus Hybrid Hook–Screw Instrumentation in the Treatment of Thoracic Adolescent Idiopathic Scoliosis (AIS): A Prospective Comparative Cohort Study. *Healthcare* **2022**, *10*, 1455. [CrossRef] [PubMed]
90. Erkilinc, M.; Coathup, M.; Liska, M.G.; Lovevoy, J. Can placement of hook at the upper instrumented level decrease the proximal junctional kyphosis risk in adolescent idiopathic scoliosis? *Eur. Spine J.* **2023**, *32*, 3113–3117. [CrossRef] [PubMed]

Disclaimer/Publisher's Note: The statements, opinions and data contained in all publications are solely those of the individual author(s) and contributor(s) and not of MDPI and/or the editor(s). MDPI and/or the editor(s) disclaim responsibility for any injury to people or property resulting from any ideas, methods, instructions or products referred to in the content.

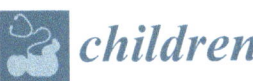

Article

Posterior Vertebral Body Tethering: A Preliminary Study of a New Technique to Correct Lenke 5C Lumbar Curves in Adolescent Idiopathic Scoliosis

Jean-Damien Metaizeau * and Delphy Denis

Department of Paediatric Orthopaedic Surgery, Chu Dijon, 21000 Dijon, France
* Correspondence: jean-damien.metaizeau@chu-dijon.fr; Tel.: +33-611939917

Abstract: Vertebral body tethering has been approved for adolescent scoliosis correction. The usual approach is anterior, which is relatively easy for the thoracic spine, but becomes much more challenging for the lumbar curves, with a higher rate of complications. The purpose of this study was to describe and evaluate the first results of a new posterior vertebral body tethering (PVBT) technique using pedicle screws through a posterolateral Wiltse approach. Twenty-two patients with 5C idiopathic scoliosis (Lenke classification) were included in this retrospective study, with a follow up of 2 years after surgery. The lumbar and thoracic curves were measured pre-operatively (POS), at first standing (FS) and at 2 years (2Y). Complications were also analysed. A significant improvement of 30.7° was observed for lumbar curve magnitude between POS and 2Y. Both the thoracic kyphosis and the lumbar lordosis remained stable. Thirteen complications were noted: three led to posterior arthrodesis, three needed a revision with a good outcome, and the seven others (overcorrections, screw breakage or pull-out) achieved a good result. PVBT seems an effective technique for the management of type 5 C adolescent idiopathic scoliosis. The complication rate seems high but is probably secondary to the learning curve of this new technic as it concerns only the first half of the patients.

Keywords: growth modulation; idiopathic scoliosis

1. Introduction

Scoliosis affects thousands of children worldwide. A curve of 45 degrees or higher is typically regarded as an indication to surgical treatment, as these curves typically continue to progress even in skeletally mature patients [1–4]. While various treatment options exist to address this condition, one innovative technique has gained increasing attention in recent years: Anterior Vertebral Body Tethering (AVBT). This surgical technique was developed for the treatment of severe scoliosis in adolescents with two main objectives: to avoid fusion and maintain spine flexibility [5–8].

It is an alternative option to Posterior Spinal Fusion (PSF), which remains the gold standard as it provides sustainable long-term outcomes, but is associated with potential long-term complications such as degenerative disc disease, back pain, radiculopathy and loss of mobility [2,9–11].

Most of the studies on anterior vertebral body tethering focus on the thoracic spine; there are very few for lumbar curves and to our knowledge, none with a posterior approach. The lumbar spine is the most mobile part of the spine, so to maintain its mobility is essential. But in these cases, surgery is more complex as a mini lumbar approach is needed; this is technically demanding, with potential complications [5,12]. Indeed, it is more difficult to put the screws in the lumbar area through the ilio-psoas muscle between nerves and vessels than in the thoracic spine, and a lot of surgeons are not used to these anterior approaches even though they are very familiar with posterior approaches.

Citation: Metaizeau, J.-D.; Denis, D. Posterior Vertebral Body Tethering: A Preliminary Study of a New Technique to Correct Lenke 5C Lumbar Curves in Adolescent Idiopathic Scoliosis. *Children* **2024**, *11*, 157. https://doi.org/10.3390/children11020157

Academic Editors: Reinald Brunner and Nathan M. Novotny

Received: 22 November 2023
Revised: 21 December 2023
Accepted: 24 January 2024
Published: 26 January 2024

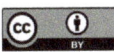

Copyright: © 2024 by the authors. Licensee MDPI, Basel, Switzerland. This article is an open access article distributed under the terms and conditions of the Creative Commons Attribution (CC BY) license (https://creativecommons.org/licenses/by/4.0/).

This is why we developed the Posterior Vertebral Body Tethering (PVBT), using the same principles; brace effect and growth modulation [1], but through a posterior Wiltse approach [13]. This makes the technique easier, with the benefit of placing the screws posteriorly, avoiding anterior screws, which could lead to a loss of lordosis.

The main aim of the study was to verify that posterior vertebral body tethering is effective in the correction of a major curve. We also wanted to evaluate the behaviour of the thoracic curves, the modifications in the sagittal plane and the complications.

2. Materials and Methods

The present retrospective study was performed between 2018 and 2022 in our institution by two senior surgeons. All families received an information letter.

2.1. Patient Selection

The inclusion criteria were:

- Diagnosis of idiopathic scoliosis from 11 to 16 years old;
- Severe progressive curves: >35°;
- Type 5C on the Lenke Classification;
- Surgical treatment using a "Posterior Vertebral Body Tethering" as described in the operative technique;
- A minimum follow-up of 2 years.

The exclusion criteria were:

- Curves other than Lenke 5C;
- Curves < 35° or >60°;
- Secondary scoliosis.

2.2. Surgical Technique

Under general anaesthesia, the patient is placed in a prone position with all support areas padded.

A Wiltse approach is used [13–15]. A midline skin incision is made, and the superficial and deep fasciae are opened longitudinally, approximately 2–3 cm laterally on the convex side. A blunt separation of the medial multifudus and the lateral longissimus is made with the fingers (Figures 1 and 2).

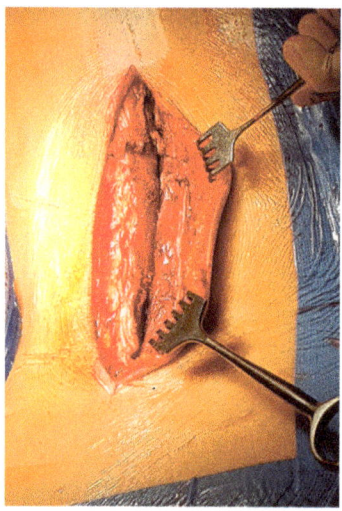

Figure 1. View of the space between the lateral longissimus and medial multifidus muscles.

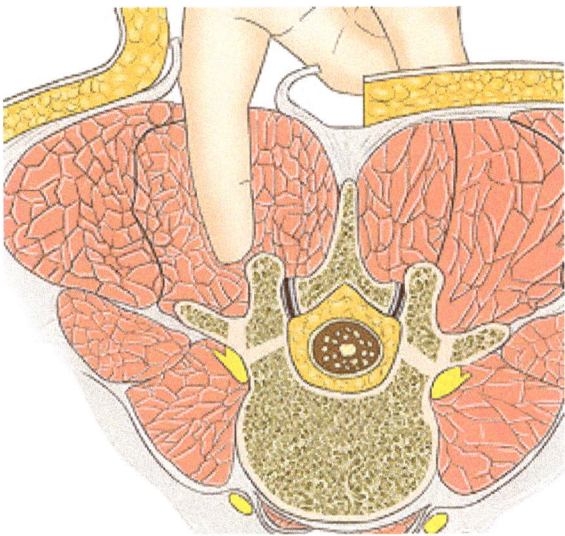

Figure 2. The space between the muscles (Ref. Ying-jie Lu, Orthopaedic Surgery [15]); it allows easy access to the joint and the transverse process.

This makes it possible to identify the transverse process and joint of each vertebra. K wire is stuck to the theoretical entry point of the screws at each level under fluoroscopy (Figures 3 and 4); note they are bent at 90° to better identify their position on the X-ray.

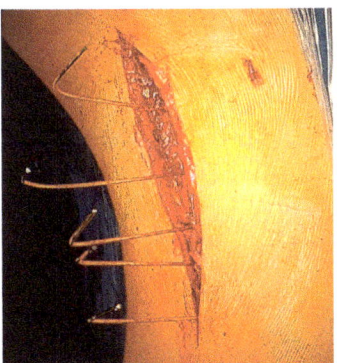

Figure 3. View of the pins: they are stuck to the theoretical entry point and bent for a better identification on the X-ray.

Then, if possible, a three-dimensional acquisition is made to evaluate the ideal path of the screws for each level. A Pediguard® is used to enter the pedicles safely and avoid the wrong way as much as possible. With a palpator, the presence of bone all around the tunnel is checked, allowing the length to also be measured. The screws (diameter 5.5 to 6.5 mm) are then put in place in the pedicles. Of course, for this step, surgeons should use the same technique they usually use for pedicle screws. Then, new fluoroscopy is performed to assess their perfect position (Figure 5).

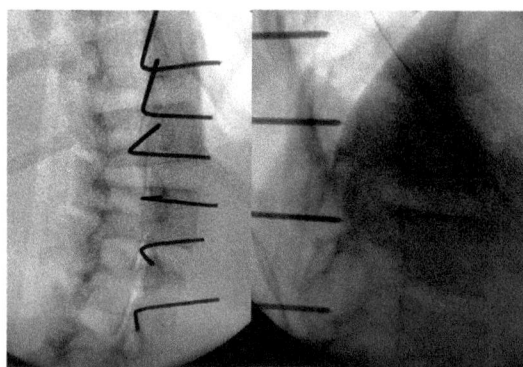

Figure 4. Frontal and sagittal view on the X-ray: it allows the perfect entry point and the right direction of the screws to be checked.

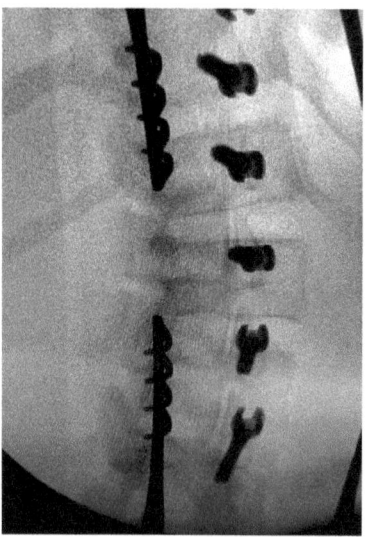

Figure 5. Frontal view of the screws; to check their good position, a sagittal view is also performed.

For those who have access, the same procedure can be carried out under navigation.

The chord is progressively placed within the screw heads from the cranial to the caudal end. Curve correction is performed with a combination of external manoeuvres (push on the convex side) and tension of the tether level by level using the appropriate tool (Figure 6).

Both fasciae are closed, the superficial fascia with the subcutaneous tissue, and then the skin with an intradermic suture. Patients walk at day 1 and are usually discharged at day 2 or 3.

The full spine when erect and the bending X-rays help to implement the right levels. The highest cranial level was T10 and the most caudal L5.

Three different types of materials were used: the CTJ+™ from NEUROFRANCE Implants® (La Ville aux Clercs, France), the BRAIVE™ from MEDTRONIC® (Minneapolis, MN, USA) and the Reflect™ from GLOBUS Medical® (Audubon, PA, USA).

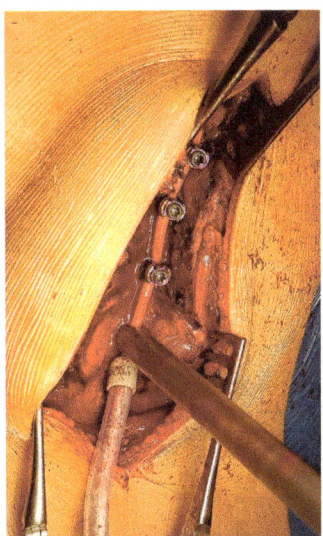

Figure 6. Tightening of the cord: the device is placed against the screws to put tension in the cable, and then the bolt is tightened. The procedure is repeated for each level.

2.3. Post-Operative Management

The first full-spine erect radiograph is performed at day 2 or 3, then at 1.5, 6, 12, 18 and 24 months post-op, and then once a year.

Sport is authorized after 6 weeks if the patients feel confident. There was no brace after surgery.

The device removal is not planned systematically, but has been carried out in some cases.

2.4. Outcomes of Interest

Baseline demographic data such as gender, age and Risser grade at surgery date were collected.

The major curve (instrumented) and compensatory curves were measured using the Cobb method, and pre-operative standing (POS), pre-operative bending for the major curve (POB), at first standing (FS) and at two years (2Y). We also evaluated thoracic kyphosis and lumbar lordosis.

The duration of hospitalisation, operative time and all the complications were recorded.

2.5. Statistical Analysis

The statistical analysis was performed with the software "BiostaTGV" (www.biostatgv.sentiweb.fr). Continuous data were expressed as mean and standard deviation, while the categorical variables were expressed as percentages. A two-sided paired t-test was performed to compare the different radiographic data. A 95% confidence interval was set for all comparisons ($p = 0.05$).

3. Results

3.1. Patient Selection and Demographic Data

During the observation period, 22 patients (16 girls and 6 boys) meeting the inclusion criteria were treated with posterior vertebral body tethering in our institution.

The mean age was 14 years old (12 to 16) and mean weight was 49 kg (35 to 64) with a Risser index of 1.5 (0 to 3).

Hospitalization stay was 3.1 days (2 to 5) and surgery time was 118 min (88 to 172).

The other data are summarized in Tables 1 and 2.

Table 1. Mean Cobb angles and sagittal angles (standard deviation).

	Pre-Operative	First Standing	Two Years
Major curve bending	15.6° (8.8)	Not applicable	Not applicable
Major curve	43.9° (9.2)	20.3° (16.2)	13.2° (28.2)
Secondary curve	29.1° (12.6)	21.9° (11.2)	19.9° (13.9)
Kyphosis (T4T12)	23.2° (7.8)	25.1° (9.5)	26.9° (12.6)
Lordosis (L1L5)	41.7° (7.8)	42.4° (10.1)	42.8° (7.5)

Table 2. Variation of lumbar Cobb angles.

	Main Curve Improvement in Percentages	Main Curve Improvement in Degrees	p Value
2Y to POB	15%	2.4°	0.96
FS to POS	54%	23.6°	0.00000002
2Y to POS	70%	30.7°	0.00005
2Y to FS	35%	7.1°	0.56

Both the major and secondary curves corrected significantly between pre-operative standing and two years: 30.7° (p = 0.00005) and 9.2° (p = 0.0013), respectively. In fact, we found the same results when comparing pre-operative standing and first standing: 23.6° (p = 0.00000002) for the major curve and 7.2° (p = 0.000102) for the secondary curve. But there was no significant difference between first standing and two years: respectively, 7.1° (p = 0.79) and 2° (p = 0.86).

The conclusion is the same when comparing pre-operative bending and first standing for the major curve: 4.7° (p = 0.96).

In the sagittal plane, the thoracic and lumbar curves did not significantly change between pre-operative standing (23.2° and 41.7°), first standing (25.1° and 42.5°) and two years (26.8° and 42.8°) (p always > 0.5).

3.2. Complications

All the complications observed and the treatments are summarised in Table 3.

Table 3. Complications.

	Number of Patients (%)	Treatment	Final Result Consequence
Pain	3 (13.6%)	1 painkiller, physiotherapy 1 screw removed (intra-canal) 1 material remove	none
Overcorrection	4 (18.1%)	1 tether section 1 posterior fusion 2 material remove	1 posterior fusion none for the others
Screw pulled out or screw breakage	4 (18.1%)	2 revisions 2 without consequence	none
Curve progression	2 (9%)	2 posterior fusion	2 posteriors fusions

Pain was considered a complication when not usual after spine surgery. One patient needed painkillers and Gabapentine®; the pain decreased with time, allowing the drugs to be stopped. The second had a typical nervous irritation which led to a CT-scan which showed an intra-canular screw in L1; the removal of the screw resolved the issue without compromising the correction. The third one had persistent pain, which did not require painkillers but was annoying; the removal of the material solved the problem.

Of the four overcorrections, one achieved a bad result with an angle of 50° and required a posterior fusion. For another, the cable was cut to stop the issue, with a good result (Cobb < 20°) at the end. Of the last two, the result at two years was good as well, and the patients asked for material removal.

Screw issues occurred in four patients: two times the proximal screws broke, and only with the CTJ+™ material from NEUROFRANCE® were there no consequences. The other two times it was the distal screws that came out; a revision was needed to put in a new screw and change the cable.

A curve progression was observed in two patients and led to a posterior fusion.

4. Discussion

The main finding of the present study is that Posterior Vertebral Body Tethering decreases the Cobb angle of the main curve of 70% (from 43.9° to 13.2°) at two years; this is similar to the average correction of the few studies on lumbar Anterior Vertebral Body Tethering: 82% for Pehlivanoglu [16] and 57% for Boeyer [5].

If we analyse the correction and look first at the results after surgery and before, there was an initial improvement of the major curve from 43.9° to 20.3° (54%) due to the "brace effect", as was observed in other studies [1]. But if we compare the results after surgery and at two years (Figure 7), it seems there was not much correction by growth modulation as described in Anterior Vertebral Body Tethering [1,17,18]. Indeed, there was an amelioration of 7.1° (35%), but it was not statistically significant. This result was unexpected, and must be investigate with studies involving more patients as there was clearly a growth modulation on several cases, leading to an overcorrection. An explanation could be the average old age of the patients with not enough growth remaining.

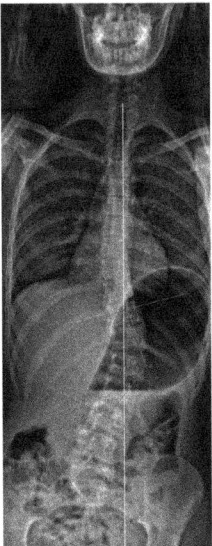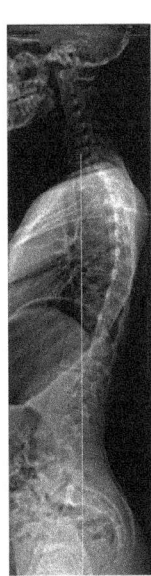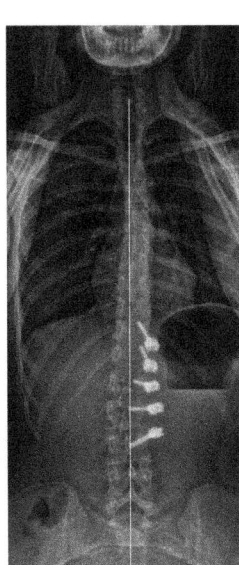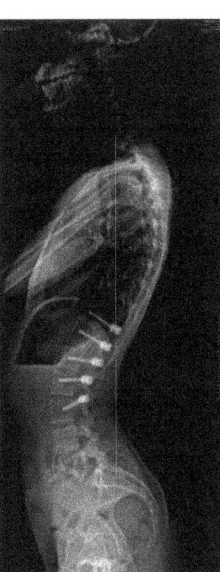

Figure 7. A 13-year-old female, Risser 0. The lumbar curve measured 38° pre-operatively, improved to −10° (slight overcorrection) at two years. In this case, there was an augmentation of both the lumbar lordosis (40° to 58°) and thoracic kyphosis (22° to 37°).

The pre-operative bending Cobb angle seems a good tool to predict the outcome of the surgery as there was no difference between the mean pre-operative bending and at two years. It also shows the importance of the flexibility of the spine in vertebral body tethering to achieve the best "brace effect" and so avoid or delay fusion [1,3].

Surprisingly, lumbar lordosis did not change as there was no difference in lumbar angles at two years and pre-operative bending. The fact that the screws are posterior would have suggested an increase in the lumbar lordosis. The thoracic kyphosis did not change, either. On this topic, studies showed a positive or neutral effect of Anterior Vertebral Body Tethering on the thoracic kyphosis [1,6,12,19,20], but we did not find any who evaluate the lumbar lordosis. Further investigations will be necessary to assess and to help understand this result. In any case, this is very interesting to know for the surgical strategy.

To our knowledge, this is the only study which evaluates lumbar vertebral body tethering using a posterior approach. The anterior approach has been described in a few studies [1,5,12,16]; it is technically demanding, and could lead to nerves issues and severe blood loss. The main operative time described in studies is 3.8 h [8], much longer than Posterior Vertebral Body Tethering, which takes about 2 h. Indeed, the technique is much easier to implement with less risk and a gentle learning curve. Moreover, all spine surgeons are used to the posterior approach, but few perform the anterior approach regularly. The length of stay was 2 to 5 days, similar to Anterior Vertebral Body Tethering [8,21].

The main advantage of vertebral body tethering is to keep spine mobility. A lot of studies demonstrate that this mobility helps to compensate sagittal issues and that a loss of lumbar mobility could lead to functional disability [11,12,16,17,22–26]. The posterior Wiltse approach respects spine mobility as much as an anterior approach.

The complication rate may seem high (59%), but only 13.6% led to a fusion; this is also probably due to the learning curves, as there was no complication for the last eight patients.

Overcorrection occurred in 18%, and is often described as common [1,3] and usually concerning the youngest patients [27]. This shows that both the brace effect and tether effect can be powerful. The brace effect seems more important in lumbar than in thoracic approaches and can lead to an overcorrection. Optimizing surgical timing will help to reduce this complication as there was no overcorrection in patient Risser 3 or higher. This can justify the cutting of the cord (one case).

In the literature, tether breakage has been reported as 2% in lumbar for Courvoisier [1], 50% at 2 years for Pehlivanoglu [16], and 71% for Baroncini [28], who also remarked that a severe and stiff pre-operative curve or a post-operative bad result led to a higher risk of tether breakage.

No tether breakage occurred in this study. The posterior position of the cable, in the main plane of mobility, could be an explanation.

The two screws that pulled out were always on the distal screws. It is very important to put in a screw as big and as long as possible to avoid this issue.

No infections were reported.

The material itself is also important. Screw breakage only occured with the CTJ+™ material from Neurofrance® and always on the proximal screw (Figure 8). Indeed, these screws had a very wide thread and a thin core, making them probably less strong for the same diameter. No breakage occurred with the Braive™ or the Reflect™ screws. Anyway, these breaks did not change the outcome of the concerned patients.

We have seen that screw issues happened at the extremities (proximal and distal). Effectively, these screws are subjected to stress in only one direction, while for the others the forces are balanced on both sides. For this reason, now we suggest adding one more vertebrae proximally and distally to serve as an anchor for the real upper or lower vertebrae and to tighten the cable gently at those levels. For example, if a T11 to L3 correction is necessary, we suggest an instrumentation from T10 to L4 with a gentle tension between T10–T11 and L3–L4.

As previously mentioned, a new surgery technique with posterior fusion has been necessary in three cases (13.6%); this rate is comparable to other studies [1,29]. In two cases, it was due to a lack of correction (Figure 9) in patients with an initial Cobb angle probably too important (>50°): this seems to be the limit for the Cobb angle for Posterior Vertebral Body Tethering unless the spine is very flexible. The other one was an overcorrection in a patient: Risser 0, Y cartilage open and a very flexible spine who was probably operated on too soon.

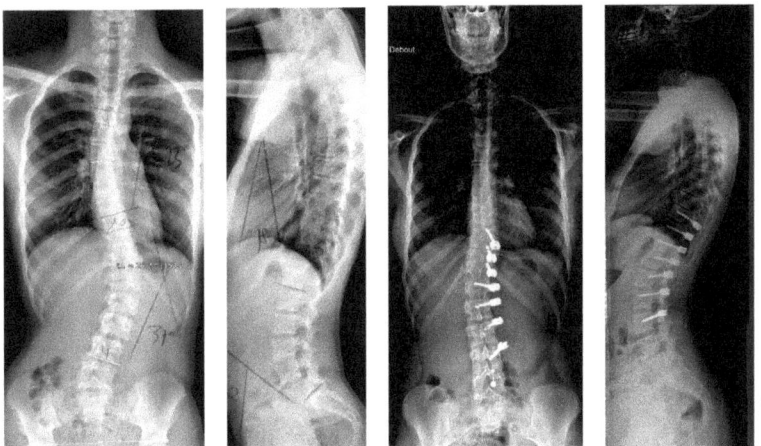

Figure 8. A 13-year-old female, Risser 2. The main curve measured 37° pre-operatively and −18° at 2 years. The overcorrection did not change the good result. In this case the secondary curve improve from 23° to 0°. Note also the broken screw.

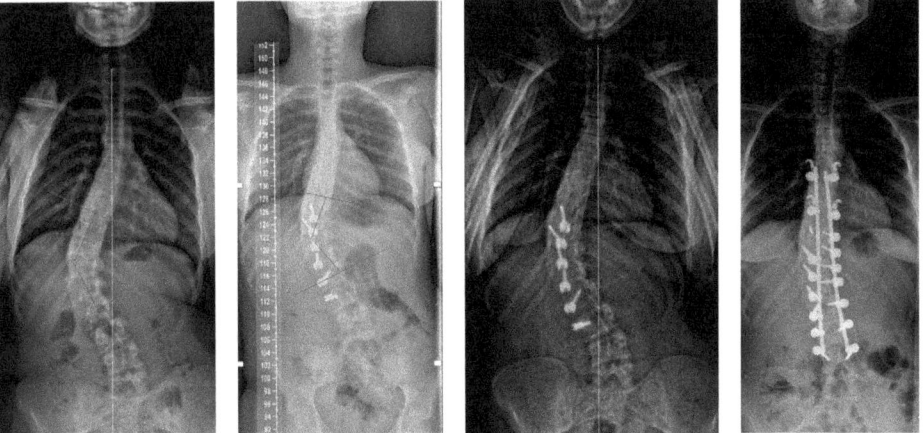

Figure 9. A 15-year-old female, Risser 3 measuring 50° pre-operatively and 44° post-operatively; became worse, requiring a posterior fusion.

We have found that if the mean angle between pre-operative bending and pre-operative standing Cobb is less than 30°, the outcome will probably be good. For example, a patient with a lumbar Cobb angle of 46° standing and 10° bending should have a good outcome ((46 + 10)/2 = 28 < 30). If this number is more than 40°, the result is less predictable. Currently, the ideal patient would be Risser 2 or more (to avoid hypercorrection) with a mean angle (as described above) under 40.

Material removal was carried out in three cases: one due to pain, and the two others at the will of the patients. We think it is possible (and probably best) to remove the material after the end of growth on all the patients with hypercorrection. In fact, in these cases, the cable has no more effect. But if there is still an angulation, the removal may not be a good idea as a loss of correction could occur after.

5. Conclusions

Posterior vertebral body tethering seems a promising technique for the treatment of type 5C lumbar adolescent idiopathic scoliosis. In our view, it is essential to keep as much spine mobility as possible, and for selected patients, it should be discussed as an alternative option before fusion. With experience, we will learn who exactly are these selected patients, and when to operate on them and so increase the efficiency of this technique. The complication rate was high but the issues were easy to resolve and became rare with experience. The new material available also helps a lot. When the technique fails and fusion is necessary, the surgery is not an issue as the spine approach will be similar.

The next step is to evaluate posterior vertebral body tethering combined with thoracic anterior vertebral body tethering for double curves (Lenke 3A or 3C) and will be the subject of another study.

Author Contributions: All authors shared all the work. All authors have read and agreed to the published version of the manuscript.

Funding: This research received no external funding.

Institutional Review Board Statement: Ethical review and approval were waived for this study after consultation of the Committee of Protection of Persons EST 1 of Dijon. This trial was outside Jarde's law field.

Informed Consent Statement: Informed consent was obtained from all the subjects involved in the study. Written informed consent has been obtained from the parents to publish this paper.

Data Availability Statement: Data are contained within the article.

Conflicts of Interest: The authors declare no conflicts of interest.

References

1. Courvoisier, A.; Baroncini, A.; Jeandel, C.; Barra, C.; Lefevre, Y.; Solla, F.; Gouron, R.; Métaizeau, J.-D.; Maximin, M.-C.; Cunin, V. Vertebral Body Tethering in AIS Management—A Preliminary Report. *Children* **2023**, *10*, 192. [CrossRef]
2. Helenius, L.; Diarbakerli, E.; Grauers, A.; Lastikka, M.; Oksanen, H.; Pajulo, O.; Löyttyniemi, E.; Manner, T.; Gerdhem, P.; Helenius, I. Back Pain and Quality of Life After Surgical Treatment for Adolescent Idiopathic Scoliosis at 5-Year Follow-up: Comparison with Healthy Controls and Patients with Untreated Idiopathic Scoliosis. *J. Bone Joint Surg. Am.* **2019**, *101*, 1460–1466. [CrossRef]
3. von Treuheim, T.D.P.; Eaker, L.; Markowitz, J.; Shankar, D.; Meyers, J.; Lonner, B. Anterior Vertebral Body Tethering for Scoliosis Patients with and without Skeletal Growth Remaining: A Retrospective Review with Minimum 2-Year Follow-Up. *Int. J. Spine Surg.* **2023**, *17*, 6–16. [CrossRef]
4. Weinstein, S.L.; Zavala, D.C.; Ponseti, I.V. Idiopathic scoliosis: Long-term follow-up and prognosis in untreated patients. *J. Bone Joint Surg. Am.* **1981**, *63*, 702–712. [CrossRef]
5. Boeyer, M.E.; Farid, S.; Wiesemann, S.; Hoernschemeyer, D.G. Outcomes of vertebral body tethering in the lumbar spine. *Spine Deform.* **2023**, *11*, 909–918. [CrossRef] [PubMed]
6. Miyanji, F.; Pawelek, J.; Nasto, L.A.; Rushton, P.; Simmonds, A.; Parent, S. Safety and efficacy of anterior vertebral body tethering in the treatment of idiopathic scoliosis. *Bone Jt. J.* **2020**, *102-B*, 1703–1708. [CrossRef] [PubMed]
7. Newton, P.O.; Bartley, C.E.; Bastrom, T.P.; Kluck, D.G.; Saito, W.; Yaszay, B. Anterior Spinal Growth Modulation in Skeletally Immature Patients with Idiopathic Scoliosis: A Comparison with Posterior Spinal Fusion at 2 to 5 Years Postoperatively. *J. Bone Joint Surg. Am.* **2020**, *102*, 769–777. [CrossRef] [PubMed]
8. Raitio, A.; Syvänen, J.; Helenius, I. Vertebral Body Tethering: Indications, Surgical Technique, and a Systematic Review of Published Results. *J. Clin. Med.* **2022**, *11*, 2576. [CrossRef] [PubMed]
9. Danielsson, A.J.; Romberg, K.; Nachemson, A.L. Spinal Range of Motion, Muscle Endurance, and Back Pain and Function at Least 20 Years after Fusion or Brace Treatment for Adolescent Idiopathic Scoliosis: A Case-Control Study. *Spine* **2006**, *31*, 275–283. [CrossRef] [PubMed]
10. Helenius, I.; Remes, V.; Yrjönen, T.; Ylikoski, M.; Schlenzka, D.; Helenius, M.; Poussa, M. Harrington and Cotrel-Dubousset Instrumentation in Adolescent Idiopathic Scoliosis: Long-Term Functional and Radiographic Outcomes. *J. Bone Jt. Surg.-Am. Vol.* **2003**, *85*, 2303–2309. [CrossRef] [PubMed]

11. Suk, S.-I.; Lee, S.-M.; Chung, E.-R.; Kim, J.-H.; Kim, S.-S. Selective thoracic fusion with segmental pedicle screw fixation in the treatment of thoracic idiopathic scoliosis: More than 5-year follow-up. *Spine* **2005**, *30*, 1602–1609. [CrossRef]
12. Trobisch, P.D.; Baroncini, A. Preliminary outcomes after vertebral body tethering (VBT) for lumbar curves and subanalysis of a 1- versus 2-tether construct. *Eur. Spine J. Off. Publ. Eur. Spine Soc. Eur. Spinal Deform. Soc. Eur. Sect. Cerv. Spine Res. Soc.* **2021**, *30*, 3570–3576. [CrossRef] [PubMed]
13. Guiroy, A.; Sícoli, A.; Masanés, N.; Ciancio, A.; Gagliardi, M.; Falavigna, A. How to perform the wiltse posterolateral spinal approach: Technical note. *Surg. Neurol. Int.* **2018**, *9*, 38. [CrossRef] [PubMed]
14. Kieser, D.C.; Thakar, C.; Cunningham, G.; Vidakovic, H.; Hammer, N.; Nnadi, C. The Value of a Modified Wiltse Approach for Deformity Correction in Neuromuscular Scoliosis. *Int. J. Spine Surg.* **2020**, *14*, 170–174. [CrossRef]
15. Lu, Y.; Miao, Y.; Zhu, T.; Wu, Q.; Shen, X.; Lu, D.; Zhu, X.; Gan, M. Comparison of the Wiltse Approach and Percutaneous Pedicle Screw Fixation Under O-arm Navigation for the Treatment of Thoracolumbar Fractures. *Orthop. Surg.* **2021**, *13*, 1618–1627. [CrossRef] [PubMed]
16. Pehlivanoglu, T.; Oltulu, I.; Erdag, Y.; Korkmaz, E.; Sarioglu, E.; Ofluoglu, E.; Aydogan, M. Double-sided vertebral body tethering of double adolescent idiopathic scoliosis curves: Radiographic outcomes of the first 13 patients with 2 years of follow-up. *Eur. Spine J. Off. Publ. Eur. Spine Soc. Eur. Spinal Deform. Soc. Eur. Sect. Cerv. Spine Res. Soc.* **2021**, *30*, 1896–1904. [CrossRef] [PubMed]
17. Newton, P.O. Spinal growth tethering: Indications and limits. *Ann. Transl. Med.* **2020**, *8*, 27. [CrossRef]
18. Newton, P.O.; Upasani, V.V.; Farnsworth, C.L.; Oka, R.; Chambers, R.C.; Dwek, J.; Kim, J.R.; Perry, A.; Mahar, A.T. Spinal growth modulation with use of a tether in an immature porcine model. *J. Bone Joint Surg. Am.* **2008**, *90*, 2695–2706. [CrossRef]
19. Cobetto, N.; Parent, S.; Aubin, C.E. 3D correction over 2years with anterior vertebral body growth modulation: A finite element analysis of screw positioning, cable tensioning and postoperative functional activities. *Clin. Biomech. Bristol. Avon. Janv.* **2018**, *51*, 26–33. [CrossRef]
20. Cobetto, N.; Aubin, C.E.; Parent, S. Anterior Vertebral Body Growth Modulation: Assessment of the 2-year Predictive Capability of a Patient-specific Finite-element Planning Tool and of the Growth Modulation Biomechanics. *Spine* **2020**, *45*, E1203–E1209. [CrossRef]
21. Mathew, S.; Larson, A.N.; Potter, D.D.; Milbrandt, T.A. Defining the learning curve in CT-guided navigated thoracoscopic vertebral body tethering. *Spine Deform.* **2021**, *9*, 1581–1589. [CrossRef] [PubMed]
22. Baroncini, A.; Trobisch, P.D.; Berrer, A.; Kobbe, P.; Tingart, M.; Eschweiler, J.; Da Paz, S.; Migliorini, F. Return to sport and daily life activities after vertebral body tethering for AIS: Analysis of the sport activity questionnaire. *Eur. Spine J. Off. Publ. Eur. Spine Soc. Eur. Spinal Deform. Soc. Eur. Sect. Cerv. Spine Res. Soc.* **2021**, *30*, 1998–2006. [CrossRef] [PubMed]
23. Buyuk, A.F.; Milbrandt, T.A.; Mathew, S.E.; Larson, A.N. Measurable Thoracic Motion Remains at 1 Year following Anterior Vertebral Body Tethering, with Sagittal Motion Greater Than Coronal Motion. *J. Bone Joint Surg. Am.* **2021**, *103*, 2299–2305. [CrossRef] [PubMed]
24. Marks, M.C.; Bastrom, T.P.; Petcharaporn, M.; Shah, S.A.; Betz, R.R.; Samdani, A.; Lonner, B.; Miyanji, F.; Newton, P.O. The Effect of Time and Fusion Length on Motion of the Unfused Lumbar Segments in Adolescent Idiopathic Scoliosis. *Spine Deform.* **2015**, *3*, 549–553. [CrossRef] [PubMed]
25. Nicolini, L.F.; Kobbe, P.; Seggewiß, J.; Greven, J.; Ribeiro, M.; Beckmann, A.; Da Paz, S.; Eschweiler, J.; Prescher, A.; Markert, B.; et al. Motion preservation surgery for scoliosis with a vertebral body tethering system: A biomechanical study. *Eur. Spine J. Off. Publ. Eur. Spine Soc. Eur. Spinal Deform. Soc. Eur. Sect. Cerv. Spine Res. Soc.* **2022**, *31*, 1013–1021. [CrossRef] [PubMed]
26. Parsch, D.; Gaertner, V.; Brocai, D.R.; Carstens, C. The effect of spinal fusion on the long-term outcome of idiopathic scoliosis. A case-control study. *J. Bone Joint Surg. Br.* **2001**, *83*, 1133–1136. [CrossRef]
27. Mariscal, G.; Morales, J.; Pérez, S.; Rubio-Belmar, P.A.; Bovea-Marco, M.; Bas, J.L.; Bas, P.; Bas, T. Meta-analysis on the efficacy and safety of anterior vertebral body tethering in adolescent idiopathic scoliosis. *Eur. Spine J.* **2023**, *32*, 140–148. [CrossRef]
28. Baroncini, A.; Trobisch, P.; Eschweiler, J.; Migliorini, F. Analysis of the risk factors for early tether breakage following vertebral body tethering in adolescent idiopathic scoliosis. *Eur. Spine J. Off. Publ. Eur. Spine Soc. Eur. Spinal Deform. Soc. Eur. Sect. Cerv. Spine Res. Soc.* **2022**, *31*, 2348–2354. [CrossRef]
29. Wu, H.-H.; Saggi, S.; Katyal, T.; Allahabadi, S.; Siu, J.; Diab, M. 167. Combined thoracic anterior and lumbar posterior tethering vs anterior vertebral body tethering: Outcomes in skeletally immature idiopathic scoliosis. *Spine J.* **2021**, *21*, S84. [CrossRef]

Disclaimer/Publisher's Note: The statements, opinions and data contained in all publications are solely those of the individual author(s) and contributor(s) and not of MDPI and/or the editor(s). MDPI and/or the editor(s) disclaim responsibility for any injury to people or property resulting from any ideas, methods, instructions or products referred to in the content.

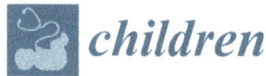

Case Report

Clinical Consequences of Unreconstructed Pelvic Defect Caused by Osteosarcoma with Subsequent Progressive Scoliosis in a Pediatric Patient—Case Report

Sławomir Zacha [1], Katarzyna Kotrych [2], Wojciech Zacha [1,*], Jowita Biernawska [3], Arkadiusz Ali [1], Dawid Ciechanowicz [3], Paweł Ziętek [3] and Daniel Kotrych [1]

1. Department of Children Orthopedics and Musculoskeletal Oncology, Pomeranian Medical University of Szczecin, 71-252 Szczecin, Poland; slawomir.zacha@pum.edu.pl (S.Z.)
2. Department of Anesthesiology and Intensive Therapy, Pomeranian Medical University of Szczecin, 71-252 Szczecin, Poland
3. Department of Orthopedics, Traumatology and Musculoskeletal Oncology, Pomeranian Medical University of Szczecin, 71-252 Szczecin, Poland
* Correspondence: wojciechzacha@gmail.com; Tel.: +48-604436990

Abstract: Osteosarcoma is the most common primary malignant bone tumor in children and adolescents. The standard and most effective treatment is wide resection of the tumor combined with neoadjuvant chemotherapy. Adolescent idiopathic scoliosis (AIS) is a genetically determined three-dimensional spinal deformity, which occurs in teenage patients and is mostly progressive. The basic management strategy is surgical treatment when the curve exceeds 50 degrees. However, the indications are different in oncologic patients. The aim of this study was to describe a case of adolescent scoliosis with osteosarcoma of the pelvis. The authors conducted a scoping review using PubMed and Embase to analyze the state of knowledge. The presented paper is the first report of pelvis osteosarcoma coexisting with adolescent idiopathic scoliosis. Treatment for this complex case finished with very good results, with no recurrence observed during the nine-year follow-up.

Keywords: adolescent idiopathic scoliosis; osteosarcoma; surgical treatment; hemipelvectomy; 3D printed implant

1. Introduction

Osteosarcoma is the most common primary malignant bone tumor in children and adolescents [1]. Its first peak of incidence occurs in patients between 15 and 25 years of age and the second peak occurs in patients above 50 years of age. The incidence rate amounts to around 0.5 to 1 per million population per year and is more common in males [2]. The most common sites of occurrence are the femur, tibia and humerus, followed by the pelvis and skull [3]. Tumors located around the pelvis and a lack of proper reconstruction of postoperative bone defects cause secondary axial skeleton deformities. Symptoms deriving from a pelvic bone sarcoma may appear late as a dull, intermittent pain after exercise, which then becomes continuous and worsens at night. Systemic symptoms, such as fever or weight loss, are rare. The basic diagnostic method is magnetic resonance imaging supported by computed tomography, and finally, biopsy [4]. The standard and most effective treatment is wide resection of the tumor combined with neoadjuvant chemotherapy [5–7].

Adolescent idiopathic scoliosis (AIS) is a genetically determined, three-dimensional spinal deformity, which occurs in teenage patients and is mostly progressive [8]. Conservative treatment of AIS aims to stop or slow down the progression of spinal deformation. Management alternatives depend on age, bone maturity, type and severity of curvature. Also, the rate of progression has a major impact on the choice of treatment [9]. Treatments include scoliosis-specific physiotherapy and bracing, which can significantly slow AIS deterioration. When the progressive spinal curvature exceeds approximately 45–50 degrees, the basic management strategy is surgical treatment [8,10]. The indications for surgical treatment are different in oncologic patients, as the problem of cancer must be solved first.

The aim of this study was to describe a case of adolescent scoliosis with osteosarcoma of the pelvis.

2. Materials and Methods

To analyze the state of knowledge about the coexistence of scoliosis and osteosarcoma of the pelvis in the pediatric population, we conducted a scoping review. The methodological framework for conducting a scoping review was based on rules proposed by Arksey and O'Malley [11]:

1. Identifying the research question: "what are the clinical consequences of unreconstructed pelvic defect caused by osteosarcoma with subsequent progressive scoliosis in a pediatric patient?". The authors analyzed the state of knowledge about the consequences of the coexistence of idiopathic scoliosis with osteosarcoma of the pelvis in the pediatric population.
2. Identifying relevant studies: Two authors analyzed data in the PubMed and Embase databases using the keywords, "pelvic osteosarcoma", "idiopathic scoliosis" and "children". A manual search for references was then performed using the eligible publications describing the clinical course of these comorbidities in children. Studies were searched for in English, with no restrictions on publication time.
3. Study selection: This involved post hoc inclusion and exclusion criteria. Study selection was performed by the first and last authors.
4. Charting the data: A data-charting form was developed and used to extract data from each study. A 'narrative review' method was used to extract process-oriented information from each study.
5. Collating, summarizing, and reporting results.

3. Results

3.1. Scoping Review

What are the clinical consequences of unreconstructed pelvic defects caused by osteosarcoma with subsequent progressive scoliosis in a pediatric patient? There are numerous scientific reports on the occurrence of scoliosis of various etiologies in children and separate reports describing cases of osteosarcoma. Searching both databases with predefined keywords, we found no articles. When we removed "idiopathic" and "children", we found one article describing a retrospective review plus two representative case reports. However, the mean age of patients was 47 years old [12,13].

3.2. Patient Presentation

We present a case of a 12-year-old female patient who, in 2008, was diagnosed with AIS (Lenke 1B-, Cobb angle 32° of thoracic curve). She was treated conservatively with only physiotherapy for 2 years. Despite the implemented treatment, progression of up to 40° of the thoracic curve was observed (Figure 1).

At that time, she started to complain of acute pain in the right hip and iliac bone, which did not subside after taking painkillers and was exacerbated during the night. Due to the presence of coexisting scoliosis, the patient was not diagnosed properly at first, as the pain was attributed to her spine condition. After consulting another orthopedic surgeon during scoliosis treatment, additional blood tests and pelvis X-rays were ordered. Results showed elevated alkaline phosphatase (ALP) and inflammation markers. By that time, the patient was having trouble walking without crutches. A physical examination revealed pain around the right sacroiliac joint without swelling and with unrestricted spine and hip range of motion.

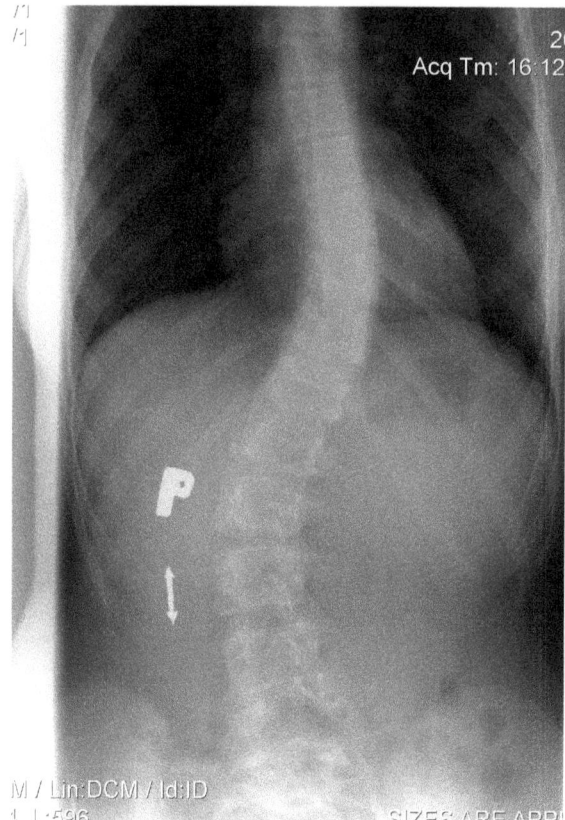

Figure 1. Lenke 1B- at the age of 14.

The patient was admitted to a medical center in Opole, Poland, in December 2012, where additional imaging was conducted. Magnetic resonance imaging (MRI) showed a tumor localized in the right iliac bone, measuring 8.6 × 7.4 × 12.5 cm in size (Figure 2). Multiple metastases in the lungs were also documented using chest computed tomography (CT). The girl was urgently transferred to the University Department of Pediatric Oncology and Bone Marrow Transplantation in Wroclaw, Poland.

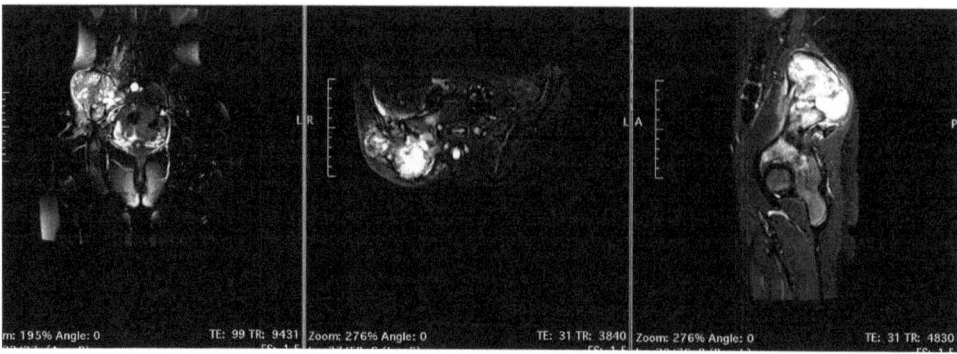

Figure 2. Osteosarcoma of the right ilium in MRI view.

3.3. Patient Management & Outcomes

3.3.1. Pelvis Osteosarcoma

Chemotherapy was administered according to protocol after the biopsy revealed the diagnosis of osteosarcoma. Due to the full remission of metastases after 10 months, hemipelvectomy with illiosacral stabilization using a plate was performed in The Department of Pediatric Surgery of Lower Silesian Specialized Hospital in Wroclaw in October 2013 (Figure 3). The histopathological test confirmed the diagnosis of osteosarcoma (high-grade, G3; mixed form; pleomorphic-like).

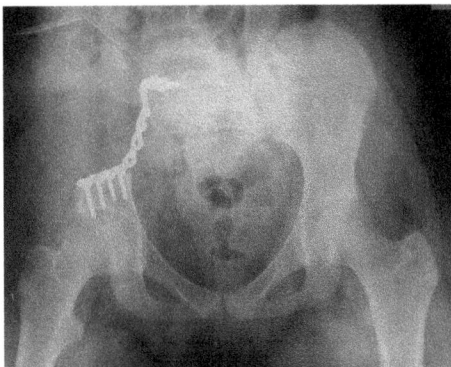

Figure 3. Postoperative X-ray.

Postoperatively, paresis of the right sciatic nerve was noticed. The resection margins were confirmed to be clear (R0). Unfortunately, the method of reconstruction used proved to be inadequate. Six weeks after surgery, the pelvis happened to break and the pelvic ring was destabilized, causing biomechanical insufficiency. For this reason, the decision was made to proceed with the next stage of surgical treatment using a similar internal fixation. It was complicated by a screw perforating into the L4/L5 intervertebral space, damaging the L4 root on the right side (Figure 4). The patient presented with severe symptoms, such as unbearable neuropathic pain, sciatic nerve palsy and complete walking disability. The patient was dismissed from the surgical department and completed complementary chemotherapy within nine months. Throughout all the periods spent under oncologic treatment, the patient was unable to walk, presented with persistent radiculopathy and a neurologic deficit, and developed depression.

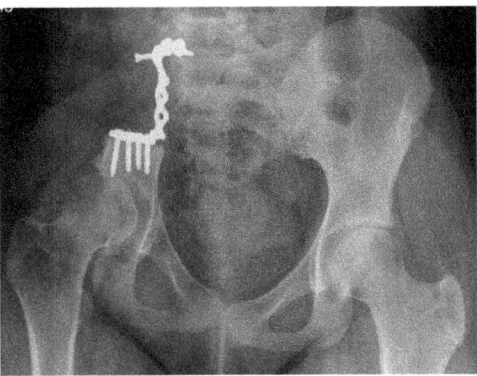

Figure 4. Breakage and destabilization of the plate.

Finally, systemic therapy had been completed. Due to the failure of the last surgical treatment, the patient was referred to another medical center specializing in cancers of the musculoskeletal system in children—Department of Orthopedics, Traumatology and Musculoskeletal Oncology in Szczecin, Poland. She was qualified for revision surgery and pelvic defect reconstruction by means of custom-made MUTARS 3D-printed endoprosthesis (Implantcast®, Hamburg, Germany). The implant design was based on 0.6 mm CT scans. The idea was not only to restore the defect, but also to support the sacrum to restore proper trunk balance (Figure 5).

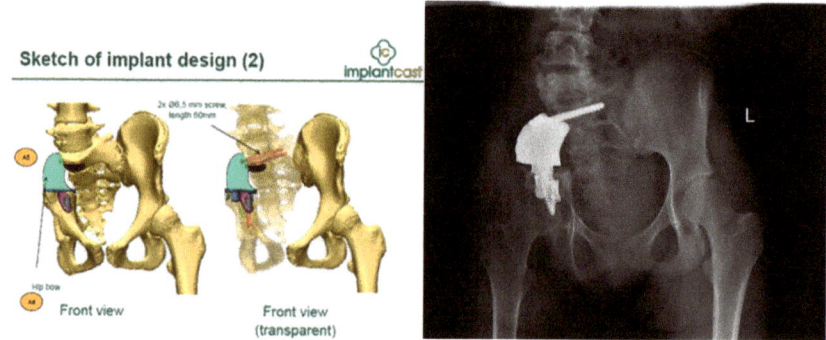

Figure 5. MUTARS 3D-printed implant design and postoperative X-ray view.

The surgery was performed in April 2015. The patient was placed in a floppy lateral position on the healthy side. An incision was made in a postoperative scar, and the broken plate was exposed and removed. The 3D-printed prosthesis was implanted and attached to the remaining iliac and sciatic bone, and to the sacrum at the level of S1 and S2 (Figure 5). There were no postoperative complications. Within the first seven days following 3D reconstruction, the pain significantly diminished to VAS 4, and the patient was able to walk alone with crutch support. Within the next six months, the sciatic nerve recovered from complete damage to 50% of its functional level. For another two years, the patient functioned well without pain and did not require pharmacological treatment.

She was in a constant rehabilitation program and under outpatient orthopedic control. Within that time, we observed substantial osseointegration of the pelvic implant, confirmed by SPECT-CT bone scintigraphy.

3.3.2. Spine Deformity

What was first a Cobb angle of 32° progressed to a Cobb angle of 68°, which required surgical intervention (Figure 6). Additionally, the curve morphology changed from double-curve Lenke 1B to a longitudinal thoracolumbar left curve due to the oblique orientation of the L4 upper endplate. At the age of 21, due to an increasing functional disorder and persistent back pain, the decision for surgical reduction of the spine was made in January 2021. The long period between the treatment of a malignant pelvic tumor and the correction of scoliosis was caused by the lack of consent for the next procedure by the patient and her family. Magnetic resonance imaging of the spine performed before spine surgery did not show any abnormalities in the neural structures.

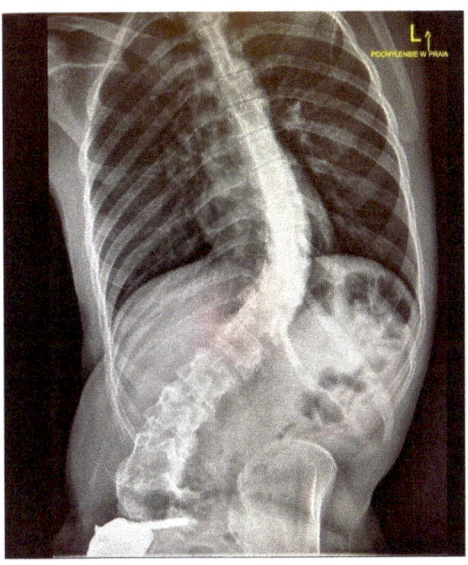

Figure 6. Progression and transformation of curve(Cobb 68°)—before surgery.

The aim of the first stage was to reduce the deformity of the lower lumbar part and to achieve a proper position of the L4 upper endplate. The procedure was performed in the Independent Public Specialized Health Care Center in Szczecin–Zdroje, Poland. The procedure involved the transpedicular fusion of L3-S2 from a posterior approach, and a lateral wedge osteotomy of L4 and L5 from an anterior approach (Medicrea®, Rillieux-la-Pape, France) (Figure 7). During the osteotomy and ossified tissue removal, the external iliac vein was damaged and repaired by a vessel surgeon, which significantly prolonged the operation to up to nine hours. The postoperative recovery period passed without complication. The patient was discharged from the hospital eleven days postoperation.

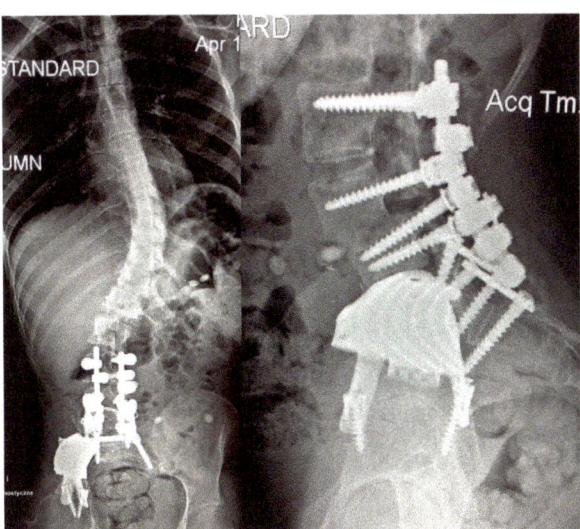

Figure 7. Surgical treatment stage one with L4 osteotomy and posterior stabilization VL3-VS2—directly after surgery.

In the second stage of surgery in December 2021, transpedicular selective reduction of Th7-L1 was performed from a posterior approach (Medicrea®, France) (Figure 8). In both stages of surgical treatment of spinal deformities, the screws were inserted using the free-hand technique. The decision to perform a selective spondylodesis leaving two free segments, L1/L2 and L2/L3, was made together with the patient and her family as a proposal to preserve mobility in the above-mentioned levels. They were informed about the risk of degenerative changes and instability, and the possible need for another stage of surgical treatment. They did not agree to fuse the entire operated spine. There were no postoperative complications. The patient was discharged from the hospital nine days postoperation.

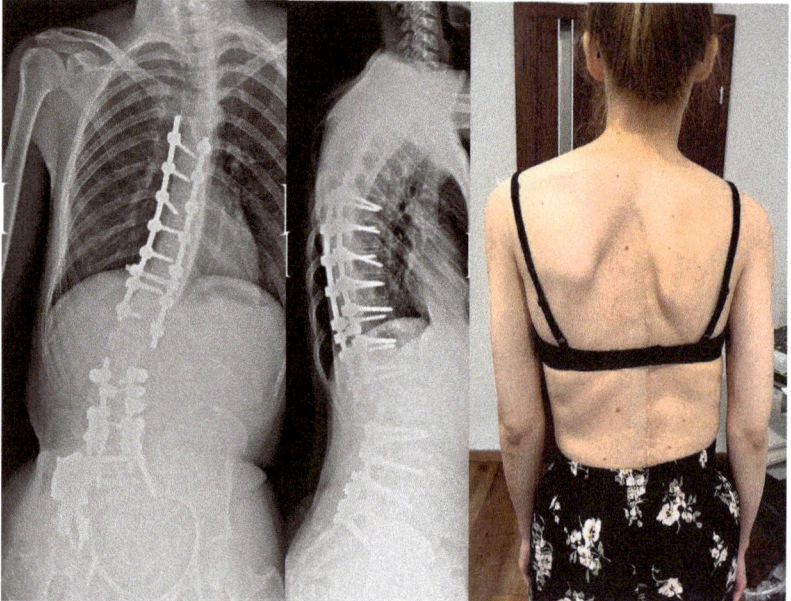

Figure 8. Surgical treatment stage two—transpedicular selective reduction of VTh7-VL1; last follow-up.

3.3.3. Clinical Outcomes

The clinical outcomes include back pain relief and further recovery from sciatic nerve palsy. After two years of rehabilitation, the patient walks with the help of crutches for longer distances and with no assistance in her flat. The persistent trunk shift visible in the X-rays was a result of right hip instability and compensation for body balance. We did not observe any deterioration in scoliosis or spinal imbalance during the follow-up. The function of the urinary bladder and anal sphincters remained intact throughout the entire treatment.

The patient is disease-free eight years after the first tumor resection and pain-free three years after scoliosis reduction. She can walk with the help of crutches for around 1000 m without stopping, and without them for around 50 m. Currently, she can perform daily activities by herself. During the last follow-up, a permanent decrease in superficial sensation on the lateral side of the right lower extremity was observed. Weakened muscle strength of the right hip abductors (Lovett 3) and right foot extensors (Lovett 3) was found according to the Lovett scale. Finally, the patient regained the ability to live independently.

4. Discussion

This presented paper is the first report of pelvis osteosarcoma coexisting with adolescent idiopathic scoliosis. Treatment of this complex case finished with fair results considering the circumstances, with no recurrence of the malignant tumor during the nine-year follow-up after pelvic reconstruction. It is necessary to point out that surgical interventions resulted in the stiffening of two extensive sections of the spine with two movable segments: L1/L2 and L2/L3. The risk for the patient is the occurrence of instability and degenerative changes in adjacent parts of the spine in the future, and the need for further surgical procedures. Moreover, the weakening of the abductor muscles of the operated hip joint and partial damage to the sciatic nerve significantly impaired the patient's walking ability.

Hemipelvectomy due to osteosarcoma is a lifesaving surgery and long-term survival is poor. The complication rate of hemipelvectomy is between 40 and 60% [14–18]. Currently, the treatment method using custom-made 3D-printed prostheses is considered a golden standard [19].

As shown by Beck et al., both internal and external hemipelvectomies were performed using different kinds of stabilization, but 3D-printed prostheses were not used.

The initial treatment of this presented case, using a plate for stabilizing the sacrum to the iliac bone, was not efficient enough. It caused an implant failure and the necessity of additional treatment. Partial sciatic nerve palsy, which occurred in our case, is often unavoidable according to the literature [20].

Sacroiliac instability is a common complication after hemipelvectomy with different stabilization implants. This biomechanical impact on spine function may cause iatrogenic deformities, which require surgical intervention [21].

There was a single case report of scoliosis operative reduction after external hemipelvectomy and one case report of scoliosis that occurred after revision surgery for pelvic reconstruction and spinopelvic fixation, in which the authors decided against operative reduction of scoliosis [12,13]. This presented case report is the first one with scoliosis reduction in a patient who previously underwent 3D reconstruction of the pelvis after hemipelvectomy. What makes this case unique is the conversion and progression of preexisting idiopathic scoliosis into an iatrogenic deformity caused by unilateral spinal fusion with the steel plate used in the first and second pelvic surgeries. Even if the scoliosis was considered idiopathic, its etiology was potentially tumor-related from the beginning.

There are not many articles describing this topic in the available literature. Using the keywords "scoliosis" and "pelvis tumors", one can find 38 items in the PubMed database. However, most of them are not relevant to our research. The vast majority of them describe the development of secondary scoliosis after pelvic ring reconstruction, postoperative development of desmoid tumors after surgical correction of adult spinal deformities, the adult population with tumors in the pelvis or degenerative scoliosis in adults. One of them describes a biomechanical study.

There are only two articles relevant to our topic. Wang et al. showed a rare case of osteoblastoma combined with a severe scoliosis deformity in a 14-year-old girl. However, the authors believed that the scoliosis deformity, pelvic obliquity and spinal imbalance were caused by this benign tumor. The patient underwent tumor excision and scoliosis correction at the same time. The patient had full neurological recovery with no aggravation of scoliosis or spinal imbalance during the follow-up [22].

Jackson and Gokaslan described the results of treatment for 13 patients who required spinal–pelvic fixation secondary to instability caused by lumbosacral neoplasms to prevent secondary scoliosis [23].

We deem our results satisfactory, all things considered. Although the radiological results of spine deformity correction are not excellent, we achieved proper cosmetic and functional results that are acceptable for both us and the patient.

5. Limitations

We acknowledge that our study had its limitations due to the incomplete radiological documentation before the final treatment. This is because the patient was treated in various medical centers in Poland initially, and we were unable to obtain all the data we needed.

Author Contributions: Conceptualization, S.Z., D.K., W.Z.; methodology, J.B.; formal analysis, S.Z., D.K., P.Z.; investigation, S.Z., D.K., P.Z.; resources, W.Z., S.Z.; data curation, S.Z., D.K., K.K.; writing—original draft preparation, W.Z., A.A., S.Z., D.C.; writing—W.Z., S.Z., J.B.; visualization, A.A., W.Z., K.K.; supervision, S.Z., D.K.; project administration, S.Z., J.B.; funding acquisition, J.B., S.Z. All authors have read and agreed to the published version of the manuscript.

Funding: This research received no external funding.

Institutional Review Board Statement: This study did not require ethical approval.

Informed Consent Statement: Informed consent was obtained from all subjects involved in the study.

Data Availability Statement: The original contributions presented in the study are included in the article, further inquiries can be directed to the corresponding author.

Conflicts of Interest: The authors declare no conflicts of interest.

References

1. Raciborska, A.; Rogowska, E. Guzy kości u dzieci i młodzieży—ważne informacje dla Pediatry. *Pediatr. Dyplom.* **2015**, *19*, 34–37.
2. Lanzkowsky, P. *Manual of Pediatric Hematology and Oncology*; Academic Press: Cambridge, MA, USA, 2005; Volume 742.
3. Ottaviani, G.; Jaffe, N. The epidemiology of osteosarcoma. *Cancer Treat. Res.* **2009**, *152*, 3–13. [PubMed]
4. Meyer, J.S.; Nadel, H.R.; Marina, N.; Womer, R.B.; Brown, K.L.B.; Eary, J.; Gorlick, R.; Grier, H.E.; Randall, R.L.; Lawlor, E.R.; et al. Imaging guidelines for children with Ewing sarcoma and osteosarcoma: A report from the children's oncology group bone tumor committee. *Pediatr. Blood Cancer* **2008**, *51*, 163–170. [CrossRef] [PubMed]
5. Geller, D.S.; Gorlick, R. Osteosarcoma: A review of diagnosis, management, and treatment strategies. *Clin. Adv. Hematol. Oncol.* **2010**, *8*, 705–718. [PubMed]
6. Brown, J.M.; Matichak, D.; Rakoczy, K.; Groundland, J. Osteosarcoma of the pelvis: Clinical presentation and overall survival. *Sarcoma* **2021**, *2021*, 8027314. [CrossRef] [PubMed]
7. Couto, A.G.; Araújo, B.; Torres de Vasconcelos, R.A.; Renni, M.J.; Da Fonseca, C.O.; Cavalcanti, I.L. Survival rate and perioperative data of patients who have undergone hemipelvectomy: A retrospective case series. *World J. Surg. Oncol.* **2016**, *14*, 255. [CrossRef]
8. Addai, D.; Zarkos, J.; Bowey, A.J. Current concepts in the diagnosis and management of adolescent idiopathic scoliosis. *Childs Nerv. Syst.* **2020**, *36*, 1111–1119. [CrossRef] [PubMed]
9. Kuznia, A.L.; Hernandez, A.K.; Lee, L.U. Adolescent Idiopathic Scoliosis: Common Questions and Answers. *Am. Fam. Physician* **2020**, *101*, 19–23. [PubMed]
10. Heyer, J.H.; Baldwin, K.D.; Shah, A.S.; Flynn, J.M. Benchmarking surgical indications for adolescent idiopathic scoliosis across time, region, and patient population: A study of 4229 cases. *Spine Deform.* **2022**, *10*, 833–840. [CrossRef]
11. Arksey, H.; O'Malley, L. Scoping studies: Towards a methodological framework. *Int. J. Soc. Res. Methodol.* **2005**, *8*, 19–32. [CrossRef]
12. Papanastassiou, I.; Boland, P.J.; Boachie-Adjei, O.; Morris, C.D.; Healey, J.H. Scoliosis after extended hemipelvectomy. *Spine* **2010**, *35*, 1328–1333. [CrossRef] [PubMed]
13. Ito, T.; Fujibayashi, S.; Otsuki, B.; Tanida, S.; Okamoto, T.; Matsuda, S. Remaining spine deformity after revision surgery for pelvic reconstruction and spinopelvic fixation: Illustrative case. *J. Neurosurg. Case Lessons* **2021**, *2*, CASE21209. [CrossRef] [PubMed]
14. Kawai, A.; Huvos, A.G.; Meyers, P.A.; Healey, J.H. Osteosarcoma of the pelvis. Oncologic results of 40 patients. *Clin. Orthop. Relat. Res.* **1998**, *348*, 196–207.
15. Senchenkov, A.; Moran, S.L.; Petty, P.M.; Knoetgen, J.; Clay, R.P.; Bite, U.; Barnes, S.A.; Sim, F.H. Predictors of complications and outcomes of external hemipelvectomy wounds: Account of 160 consecutive cases. *Ann. Surg. Oncol.* **2008**, *15*, 355–363. [CrossRef] [PubMed]
16. Apffelstaedt, J.P.; Driscoll, D.L.; Spellman, J.E.; Velez, A.F.; Gibbs, J.F.; Karakousis, C.P. Complications and outcome of external hemipelvectomy in the management of pelvic tumors. *Ann. Surg. Oncol.* **1996**, *3*, 304–309. [CrossRef] [PubMed]
17. Shin, K.H.; Rougraff, B.T.; Simon, M.A. Oncologic outcomes of primary bone sarcomas of the pelvis. *Clin. Orthop. Relat. Res.* **1994**, *304*, 207–217. [CrossRef]
18. Beck, L.A.; Einertson, M.J.; Winemiller, M.H.; DePompolo, R.W.; Hoppe, K.M.; Sim, F.F. Functional Outcomes and Quality of Life After Tumor-Related Hemipelvectomy. *Phys. Ther.* **2008**, *88*, 916–927. [CrossRef] [PubMed]
19. Liang, H.; Ji, T.; Zhang, Y.; Wang, Y.; Guo, W. Reconstruction with 3D-printed pelvic endoprostheses after resection of a pelvic tumor. *Bone Joint J.* **2017**, *99-B*, 267–275. [CrossRef]
20. Barrientos-Ruiz, I.; Ortiz-Cruz, E.J.; Peleteiro-Pensado, M. Reconstruction After Hemipelvectomy With the Ice-Cream Cone Prosthesis: What Are the Short-term Clinical Results? *Clin. Orthop. Relat. Res.* **2017**, *475*, 735–741. [CrossRef]
21. Zavras, A.G.; Fice, M.P.; Dandu, N.; Munim, M.A.; Colman, M.W. Comparison of Reconstruction Techniques Following Sacroiliac Tumor Resection: A Systematic Review. *Ann. Surg. Oncol.* **2022**, *29*, 7081–7091. [CrossRef]

22. Wang, L.N.; Hu, B.W.; Wang, L.; Yang, X.; Liu, L.M.; Song, Y.M. A rare case of osteoblastoma combined with severe scoliosis deformity, coronal and sagittal imbalance. *BMC Musculoskelet. Disord.* **2017**, *18*, 538. [CrossRef] [PubMed]
23. Jackson, R.J.; Gokaslan, Z.L. Spinal-pelvic fixation I n patient with lumbosacral neoplasms. *J. Neurosurg.* **2000**, *92* (Suppl. S1), 61–70. [CrossRef] [PubMed]

Disclaimer/Publisher's Note: The statements, opinions and data contained in all publications are solely those of the individual author(s) and contributor(s) and not of MDPI and/or the editor(s). MDPI and/or the editor(s) disclaim responsibility for any injury to people or property resulting from any ideas, methods, instructions or products referred to in the content.

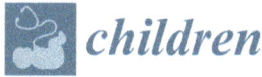

Systematic Review

Ponte Osteotomies in the Surgical Treatment of Adolescent Idiopathic Scoliosis: A Systematic Review of the Literature and Meta-Analysis of Comparative Studies

Cesare Faldini [1,2,*], Giovanni Viroli [1,2], Matteo Traversari [1,2], Marco Manzetti [1,2], Marco Ialuna [1,2], Francesco Sartini [1,2], Alessandro Cargeli [1,2], Stefania Claudia Parisi [1,2] and Alberto Ruffilli [1,2]

[1] Department of Biomedical and Neuromotor Science—DIBINEM, University of Bologna, 40126 Bologna, Italy; giovanni.viroli@ior.it (G.V.); matteo.traversari@ior.it (M.T.); marco.manzetti@ior.it (M.M.); marco.ialuna@ior.it (M.I.); francesco.sartini@ior.it (F.S.); alessandro.cargeli@ior.it (A.C.); stefaniaclaudia.parisi@ior.it (S.C.P.); alberto.ruffilli@ior.it (A.R.)
[2] 1st Orthopaedic and Traumatologic Clinic, IRCCS Istituto Ortopedico Rizzoli, 40136 Bologna, Italy
* Correspondence: cesare.faldini@ior.it

Citation: Faldini, C.; Viroli, G.; Traversari, M.; Manzetti, M.; Ialuna, M.; Sartini, F.; Cargeli, A.; Parisi, S.C.; Ruffilli, A. Ponte Osteotomies in the Surgical Treatment of Adolescent Idiopathic Scoliosis: A Systematic Review of the Literature and Meta-Analysis of Comparative Studies. *Children* **2024**, *11*, 92. https://doi.org/10.3390/children11010092

Academic Editors: Federico Solla and Luigi Aurelio Nasto

Received: 21 December 2023
Revised: 9 January 2024
Accepted: 10 January 2024
Published: 12 January 2024

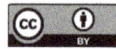

Copyright: © 2024 by the authors. Licensee MDPI, Basel, Switzerland. This article is an open access article distributed under the terms and conditions of the Creative Commons Attribution (CC BY) license (https://creativecommons.org/licenses/by/4.0/).

Abstract: The purpose of the present paper is to assess if Ponte osteotomies (POs) allow for a better correction in adolescent idiopathic scoliosis (AIS) surgery and to investigate their safety profile. A systematic search of electronic databases was conducted. Inclusion criteria: comparative studies that reported the outcomes of AIS patients who underwent surgical correction through posterior-only approach with and without POs. Clinical and radiographic outcomes were extracted and summarized. Meta-analyses were performed to estimate the differences between patients treated with and without POs. $p < 0.05$ was considered significant. In total, 9 studies were included. No significant difference in thoracic kyphosis (TK) change between patients treated with and without POs was found (+3.8°; $p = 0.06$). Considering only hypokyphotic patients, a significant difference in TK change resulted in POs patients (+6.6°; $p < 0.01$), while a non-significant TK change resulted in normokyphotic patients (+0.2°; $p = 0.96$). No significant difference in coronal correction (2.5°; $p = 0.10$) was recorded. Significant estimated blood loss (EBL) (142.5 mL; $p = 0.04$) and surgical time (21.5 min; $p = 0.04$) differences were found with POs. Regarding complications rate, the meta-analysis showed a non-significant log odds ratio of 1.1 ($p = 0.08$) with POs. In conclusion, POs allow for the restoration of TK in hypokyphotic AIS, without a significantly greater TK change in normokyphotic patients, nor a significantly better coronal correction. Considering the significantly greater EBL and the trend toward a higher complications rate, the correct indication for POs is crucial.

Keywords: adolescent idiopathic scoliosis; AIS; Ponte osteotomies; posterior column osteotomies; deformity correction

1. Introduction

Adolescent idiopathic scoliosis (AIS) surgery, during the past 20 years, has experienced major advancements. More specifically, the wide spread of modern pedicle fixation systems, along with the development of powerful corrective techniques such as direct vertebral rotation (DVR), has enabled powerful posterior-only corrective surgeries, especially in the coronal and axial planes. Conversely, considering the tridimensional nature of AIS, the results of surgical correction on the sagittal plane component of the deformity, typically characterized by a reduction in thoracic kyphosis (TK) due to anterior spinal overgrowth [1], have been inconsistent [2]. In particular, several studies have demonstrated not only a failure in the restoration of TK, but also a proper iatrogenic hypokyphotic effect, which has been ascribed to DVR at times [3–5] and to all-pedicle-screws-based constructs [6,7]. This aspect of AIS surgery has received growing attention since thoracic hypokyphosis is related to long term consequences in the adjacent spinal regions. In particular, Bernstein et al. [8] reported an increased risk of lumbar degenerative disc disease in patients in which TK restoration was ineffective, while Hwang et al. [9] correlated the lack of TK restoration to an increased risk of cervical spine decompensation in kyphosis after AIS surgery.

Many authors [10,11] have therefore adopted ancillary procedures such as Ponte osteotomies (POs) in order to restore TK, or at least to optimize the corrective maneuver, trying to avoid the risk of iatrogenic hypokyphosis as much as possible. Ponte osteotomies were first developed in 1987 by Alberto Ponte for the surgical correction of rigid hyperkyphosis [12]. In particular, the original technique requires a wide multilevel posterior release with the removal of all posterior column ligaments, a superior and inferior laminectomy, and a bilateral extended facetectomy. This results in substantial posterior column shortening when the osteotomy is closed. However, scoliosis correction requires an opposite effect: an elongation of the posterior column in order to restore TK in hypokyphotic scoliosis or to avoid iatrogenic hypokyphosis in normokyphotic curves. This conceptual contradiction has added to the scepticism regarding the efficacy of POs in scoliosis surgery, especially considering that POs are not risk-free.

Through a systematic literature research and a meta-analysis of comparative studies, the first aim of the present paper is to assess whether the adoption of POs allows for the restoration of TK during AIS correction surgery. The second objective is to assess the influence of POs on the coronal correction rate. The final endpoint is to determine if the use of POs results in significantly increased blood loss, operative time, and complication rate, such that their adoption for a better correction may not be justified by their safety profile.

2. Materials and Methods

A systematic review of the literature regarding the effect of POs on thoracic kyphosis as accessory procedures of surgical treatment of AIS was conducted in accordance with the PRISMA guidelines (preferred reporting items of systematic reviews) [13].

2.1. Eligibility Criteria

Only peer-reviewed publications were considered for inclusion. Studies were included if they compared the outcomes of patients affected by AIS who underwent surgical correction through a posterior-only approach with and without Ponte osteotomies. Articles in English which met the PICO (Population, Intervention, Comparison, and Outcomes) criteria on systematic reviews were considered for inclusion.

Only randomized controlled trials (RCTs) and prospective and retrospective comparative cohort studies (PCS and RCS) were considered for inclusion. In vitro studies and animal model studies were excluded, as well as case reports and case series.

2.2. Search Strategy

Studies eligible for this systematic review were identified through an electronic systematic search of PubMed and Cochrane Central Registry of Controlled Trials papers published from 2000 to May 2023.

The following search strings were used:
- (adolescent AND idiopathic AND scoliosis) OR (AIS) AND (ponte OR (ponte AND osteotomy) OR (ponte AND osteotomies) OR (multiple AND asymmetric AND ponte AND osteotomies) OR MAPO);
- ((scoliosis AND adolescent) OR AIS)) and (ponte OR (ponte AND osteotomy) OR (ponte AND osteotomies) OR MAPO OR (posterior AND column AND osteotomies) OR (posterior AND column AND osteotomy) OR (PCO)).

2.3. Study Selection

Articles considered relevant by electronic search were retrieved in full-text, and a hand-search of their bibliography was performed in order to find further related articles. Reviews and meta-analyses were also analysed to identify potentially missed eligible papers. Duplicates were removed. The study selection process was carried out in accordance with the PRISMA flowchart (Figure 1). The systematic review was not prospectively registered.

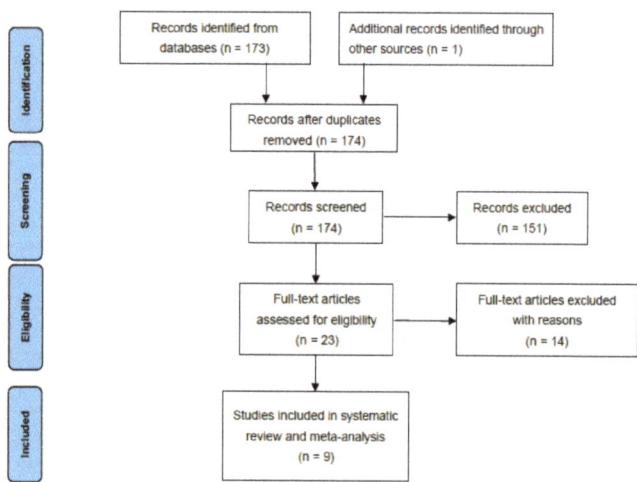

Figure 1. Prisma flowchart.

The quality of the included studies was evaluated using the Robins-I tool [14] (Figure 2).

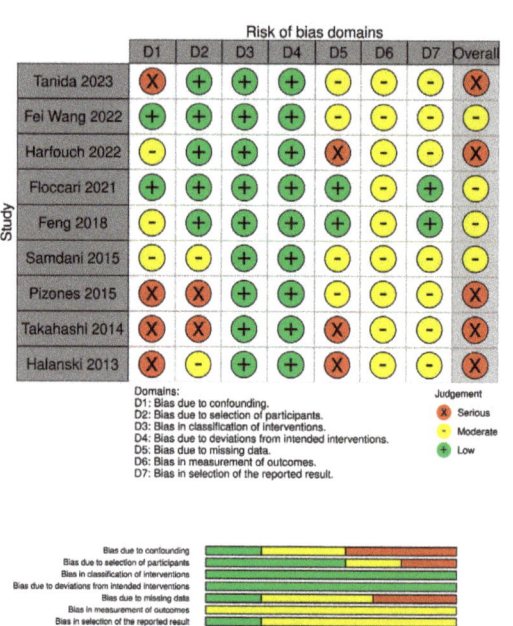

Figure 2. Risk of bias assessment according to Robins-I tool [15–23].

2.4. Data Collection Process

All included studies were analysed, and data related to baseline characteristics (Table 1) and outcomes of interest (Table 2) were extracted and summarized.

Table 1. Summary of baseline characteristics of the included studies. (AIS: adolescent idiopathic scoliosis; POs: Ponte osteotomies; PSF: posterior spinal fusion).

Author	Study Design	Level of Evidence	Patients N° (M/F)	Inclusion Criteria	Mean Patient Age (Years)	Lenke Types	Mean Risser Sign	Internal Fixation System	Posterior Release	Number of POs
Tanida 2023 (P) [22]	Retrospective comparative cohort study	III	19 (3/16)	AIS patients with Lenke 1 or 2 patterns, who underwent PSF	15.4 ± 2.8	I: 6 II: 13	/	Pedicle screws and rods	T6/7, 7/8, and 8/9 Ponte osteotomies	3
Tanida 2023 (C) [22]			18 (4/14)		15.6 ± 2.2	I: 7 II: 11	/			0
Fei Wang 2022 (P) [17]	Retrospective comparative cohort study	III	40 (4/36)	AIS patients < 18 years old, main thoracic curve > 40°, thoracic kyphosis (T5–T12) < 10°	14.50 ± 1.77	I: 40 (IA: 26, IB: 10, IC: 4)	3.80 ± 0.8	Pedicle screws and rods	Peri-apical Ponte osteotomies	3
Fei Wang 2022 (C) [17]			40 (2/38)		15.13 ± 1.57	I: 40 (IA: 18, IB: 16, IC: 6)	4.00 ± 0.8		/	0
Harfouch 2022 (P) [16]	Retrospective comparative cohort study	III	40 (8/32)	Consecutive patients affected by AIS and treated with PSF	16.7 ± 3.4	I: 14 II: 12 III: 7 IV: 5 V: 0 VI: 2	/	Pedicle screws and rods	Peri-apical Ponte osteotomies	4–6
Harfouch 2022 (C) [16]			40 (6/34)		16.1 ± 2.6	I: 15 II: 12 III: 5 IV: 4 V: 0 VI: 4	/		/	0
Floccari 2021 (P) [18]	Prospective comparative matched cohort study	III	34 (8/26)	AIS patients treated with PSF and receiving at least 2 POs, matched with analogous group who underwent PSF without the use of POs	14.6 ± 2.3	I: 11 (IA: 6, IB: 5) II: 16 (IIA: 13, IIB: 2, IIC: 1) III: 4 (IIIC: 4) VI: 3	/	Pedicle screws and rods	Peri-apical Ponte osteotomies	3.5 (2–9)
Floccari 2021 (C) [18]			34 (8/26)		14.8 ± 2.0	I: 11 (IA: 6, IB: 5) II: 16 (IIA: 13, IIB: 2, IIC: 1) III: 4 (IIIC: 4) VI: 3	/		/	0

Table 1. Cont.

Author	Study Design	Level of Evidence	Patients N° (M/F)	Inclusion Criteria	Mean Patient Age (Years)	Lenke Types	Mean Risser Sign	Internal Fixation System	Posterior Release	Number of POs
Feng 2018 (P) [19]	Retrospective comparative cohort study	III	32 (10/22)	AIS patients affected by Lenke 1-4 curves treated with PSF	15.1 ± 1.9	Lenke types 1-4, details not mentioned	3.30 ± 0.90	Pedicle screws and rods	Multilevel Ponte osteotomies (at each segment of the thoracic curve)	/
Feng 2018 (C) [19]			33 (10/23)		15.7 ± 1.9		3.10 ± 1.0		Soft tissues release	0
Samdani,2015 (P) [20]	Retrospective comparative cohort study	III	125 (27/98)	Prospective consecutive patients affected by Lenke 1A and 1B curves treated with PSF with at least 2 years of follow up	14.8 ± 2.3	I: 127 (IA: 91, IB:34)	/	Pedicle screws and rods	Ponte osteotomies	4.3 ± 1.5
Samdani, 2015 (C) [20]			66 (10/56)		14.6 ± 2.1	I: 56 (IA: 50, IB: 16)	/		Partial facetectomies with removal of inferior articular facets	0
Pizones 2015 (P) [23]	Historically controlled cohort study	III	43 (9/34)	Prospective series of patients affected by thoracic AIS who underwent PSF with POs compared with historical series of patients who underwent PSF alone	14.9 ± 2.1	I-IV (not mentioned details)	/	Sublaminar wires and hybrid instrumentation	Ponte osteotomies	/
Pizones 2015 (C) [23]			30 (5/25)		15.2 ± 2.3	I-IV (not mentioned details)	/		Not mentioned	0
Takahashi 2014 (P) [21]	Retrospective comparative cohort study	III	17 (0/17)	Patients affected by AIS who underwent skip pedicle screw fixation with POs compared with patients who underwent skip pedicle screw fixation	15.6 ± 2.0	I: 11 II: 3 IV: 1 VI: 2	/	Skip pedicle screw fixation and rods	Ponte osteotomies	3.8 ± 1.3
Takahashi 2014 (C) [21]			21 (0/21)		14.4 ± 2.5	I: 15 II: 4 VI: 2	/		Partial facetectomies with removal of inferior articular facets	0
Halanski 2013 (P) [15]	Retrospective comparative cohort study	III	17 (5/12)	Consecutive patients affected by AIS with Lenke I or II curves treated with PSF	13.2 ± 3.0	/	/	Pedicle screws and rods	Ponte osteotomies	/
Halanski 2013 (C) [15]			18 (2/16)		13.7 ± 2.0	/	/		Partial facetectomies with removal of inferior articular facets	0

Table 2. Summary of reported outcomes of the included studies. (POs: Ponte osteotomies; TK: thoracic kyphosis; IONM: intraoperative neuromonitoring; PSF: posterior spinal fusion).

Author	Mean Pre-Operative Major Cobb Angle (°)	Mean Flexibility Index of Major Curve (%)	Mean Post-Operative Major Cobb Angle (°)	Mean Correction Rate (%)	Mean Pre-Operative TK (°)	Mean Post-Operative TK (°)	Mean TK Change (°)	Mean Surgical Time (min)	Mean Intraoperative Blood Loss (mL)	Mean Length of Stay (Days)	Complication Rate (%)
Tanida 2023 (P) [22]	59.7 ± 10.3	45.5 ± 10.1	21.0 ± 6.2	64.4 ± 10.2	17.3 ± 12.7	30.7 ± 6.4	13.8 ± 9.6	368.2 ± 54.5	619.7 ± 288.0	/	/
Tanida 2023 (C) [22]	53.1 ± 5.8	38.7 ± 15.9	20.6 ± 5.3	61.0 ± 10.3	11.6 ± 10.5	22.3 ± 4.7	7.8 ± 8.0	339.8 ± 49.7	723.9 ± 285.4	/	/
Fei Wang 2022 (P) [17]	48.10 ± 3.9	/	15.18 ± 2.8	/	5.3 ± 3.2	24.23 ± 2.7	18.93	262.0 ± 28.8	1103.2 ± 115.1	/	2 (5%) (2 infections)
Fei Wang 2022 (C) [17]	50.03 ± 4.9	/	20.33 ± 3.8	/	6.45 ± 2.9	19.93 ± 2.4	13.48	229.5 ± 26.8	979.8 ± 171.7	/	1 (2.5%) (1 case of abdominal pain treated with gastrointestinal decompression)
Harfouch 2022 (P) [16]	67.5 ± 19.5	/	20.4 ± 12.5	71.0 ± 10.9	29.0 ± 13.1	25.2 ± 6.0	−3.8 ± 11.6	/	/	/	5 (12.5%) (all IONM changes, 2 cases required two-stage surgery with temporary rod)
Harfouch 2022 (C) [16]	68.1 ± 14.9	/	25.0 ± 11.1	64.2 ± 11.5	36.2 ± 14.9	17.5 ± 9.4	−18.6 ± 10.1	/	/	/	0
Floccari 2021 (P) [18]	74.5 ± 15.2	39.6 ± 12.7	29.1 ± 8.6	66.6 ± 14.1	28.0 ± 16.0	22.6 ± 8.9	−5.5 ± 14.0	296.0 ± 64.0	825.0 ± 511.1	4.4 ± 1.0	11 (32.4%) (of whom 5 were IONM critical changes, 6 reoperations for mechanical failures or infections)
Floccari 2021 (C) [18]	70.8 ± 13.4	39.1 ± 10.6	21.3 ± 9.5	58.7 ± 10.3	27.6 ± 14.5	24.6 ± 9.7	−3.0 ± 12.1	286.3 ± 63.8	861.2 ± 583.4	4.6 ± 1.4	2 (5.9%) (1 reoperation for mechanical failure, 1 for infection)
Feng 2018 (P) [19]	57.6 ± 10.3	/	19.9 ± 1.6	63.9 ± 4.5	N (18): 21.3 ± 6.7 HyperK (3): 45.3 ± 5.5 HypoK (11): 7.3 ± 1.9	N (18): 28.4 ± 4.6 HyperK (3): 27.0 ± 2.0 HypoK (11): 18.4 ± 3.2	N (18): 7.1 ± 10.3 HyperK (3): −18.3 ± 2.5 HypoK (11): 11.1 ± 2.9	243.0 ± 12.0	952.0 ± 124.0	/	1 (3.1%) (hemopneumothorax)

Table 2. Cont.

Author	Mean Pre-Operative Major Cobb Angle (°)	Mean Flexibility Index of Major Curve (%)	Mean Post-Operative Major Cobb Angle (°)	Mean Correction Rate (%)	Mean Pre-Operative TK (°)	Mean Post-Operative TK (°)	Mean TK Change (°)	Mean Surgical Time (min)	Mean Intraoperative Blood Loss (mL)	Mean Length of Stay (Days)	Complication Rate (%)
Feng 2018 (C) [19]	56.1 ± 8.9	/	19.6 ± 2.9	65.2 ± 2.4	N (19): 23.7 ± 5.5 HyperK (4): 43.0 ± 1.4 HypoK (11): 8.0 ± 1.4	N (19): 24.4 ± 6.2 HyperK (4): 30.5 ± 1.3 HypoK (11): 11.5 ± 2.4	N (19): 0.7 ± 4.6 HyperK (4): −12.5 ± 1.3 HypoK (11): 3.5 ± 2.2	196.0 ± 10.0	772.0 ± 65.0	/	2 (6.1%) (surgical site infections)
Samdani, 2015 (P) [20]	51.5 ± 8.6	47.3 ± 22.1	16.8 ± 6.3	67.1 ± 11.8	18.7 ± 13.0	21.8 ± 7.9	3.0 ± 11.6	277.4 ± 98.9	970.1 ± 566.5	5.3 ± 1.2	/
Samdani, 2015 (C) [20]	50.8 ± 8.1	54.5 ± 22.8	19.4 ± 7.0	61.8 ± 12.6	23.2 ± 12.3	22.8 ± 9.4	−0.4 ± 9.9	295.9 ± 136.4	778.9 ± 726.1	5.3 ± 1.2	/
Pizones 2015 (P) [23]	60.0 ± 9.9	/	17.4 ± 7.5	/	All cohort (43): 23.7 ± 13.7 N (27): 26 ± 6.1 HyperK (4): 52.2 ± 5.6 HypoK (12): 6.4 ± 2	All cohort: 22.0 ± 6.4 N (27): 25.9 ± 6 HyperK (4): 30.5 ± 8.5 HypoK (12): 21.3 ± 5.8	All cohort: −1.4 ± 12.5 N (27): 0.1 ± 6.9 HyperK (4): −21.7 ± 9.1 HypoK (12): 15.5 ± 7.5	258.0 ± 42.0	/	14	/
Pizones 2015 (C) [23]	60.4 ± 10.0	/	26.5 ± 8.0	/	All cohort (30): 23.5 ± 11.8 N (20): 24.2 ± 7.9 HyperK (3): 46 ± 3.4 HypoK (7): 9.8 ± 0.3	All cohort: 24.9 ± 9.9 N (20): 27.9 ± 7.5 HyperK (3): 38.5 ± 9.1 HypoK (7): 15 ± 7	All cohort: 1.0 ± 6.1 N (20): 3.4 ± 7.2 HyperK (3): −6.5 ± 5 HypoK (7): 5.6 ± 7.9	276.0 ± 54.0	/	6.7	/
Takahashi 2014 (P) [21]	52.5 ± 10.4	31.7 ± 13.2	18.4 ± 1.6	62.0 ± 2.5	11.3 ± 11.2	21.8 ± 1.7	10.5 ± 2.4	236.0 ± 13.0	1141.0 ± 150.0	/	/
Takahashi 2014 (C) [21]	51.5 ± 9.2	45.1 ± 12.3	17.8 ± 1.0	63.6 ± 2.5	13.0 ± 9.0	24.2 ± 1.9	11.2 ± 1.9	187.0 ± 9.0	745.0 ± 120.0	/	/
Halanski 2013 (P) [15]	59.0 ± 10.0	33.0 ± 19.0	9.0 ± 6.0	84.0 ± 9.0	20.0 ± 15.0	28.0 ± 8.0	8.0 ± 11.0	/	/	/	1 (5.9%) (pneumothorax)
Halanski 2013 (C) [15]	52.0 ± 8.0	41.0 ± 16.0	9.0 ± 4.0	83.0 ± 6.0	24.0 ± 12.0	25.0 ± 7.0	1.0 ± 10.0	/	/	/	1 (5.6%) (mispositioned screw that was removed)

Meta-analyses were performed when there were at least three studies to be compared. Heterogeneity between studies was assessed using the inconsistency statistic ($I^2 > 75\%$ was considered to be high heterogeneity). Publication bias was assessed with Egger's test and represented with forest plots. Standardized mean differences were used as measures of effect size. The random effect model was applied. A p-value < 0.05 was considered to be significant. All statistical analyses were conducted with Jamovi version 2.2 (The Jamovi project, Sydney, Australia) software.

3. Results

3.1. Baseline Studies Characteristics and Quality Assessment

A total of 174 studies were found through electronic search; after screening, 9 studies (1 prospective comparative matched cohort study (PCS), 1 historically controlled cohort study (HCCS), and 7 retrospective comparative cohort studies (RCS) were included. Meta-analysis was conducted on comparative studies. The risk of bias in the papers is reported in Figure 2.

A total of 667 patients were included. The mean age at surgery ranged from 13.2 ± 3.0 [15] to 16.7 ± 3.4 years [16]. Lenke type was reported for 486 patients: 353 Lenke 1 (72.6%), 87 Lenke 2 (17.9%), 20 Lenke 3 (4.1%), 10 Lenke 4 (2.1%), and 16 Lenke 6 (3.3%). As for constructs, 8 authors used all pedicle screws constructs [15–22], while one preferred hybrid constructs [23]. As for Ponte osteotomies, most authors performed a variable number of periapical osteotomies ranging from 2 to 9 [18].

3.2. Thoracic Kyphosis Change

The mean pre-operative thoracic kyphosis (T5–T12) varied from $5.3 \pm 3.2°$ [17] to $36.2 \pm 14.9°$ [16]. The mean thoracic kyphosis change after surgery ranged between $-5.5°$ [18] to $18.9°$ [17] for POs groups and from $-18.6°$ [16] to $13.5°$ [17] after posterior spinal fusion (PSF) without POs. Harfouch et al. [16] reported a larger difference in TK between patients treated with and without POs, reporting $3.8°$ of TK loss after PSF with POs and $18.6°$ of kyphosis loss after PSF without POs ($p < 0.001$). No significant difference in TK change between PSF with and without POs was found in the meta-analysis, with an estimated average mean difference of $+3.8°$ (95% CI: -0.1644 to $7.7319°$; $p = 0.0603$) (Figure 3A). No publication bias (t = 0.393, $p = 0.694$ (Figure 3B) was found, but substantial heterogeneity among studies was calculated ($I^2 = 93.5303\%$, $p < 0.0001$).

A subgroup meta-analysis was performed in order to assess the mean TK change considering only hypokyphotic patients (Lenke sagittal modifier = TK < 10°). In this, three studies were included, and POs provided a significant estimated average TK increase in this subset of patients ($+6.6°$; 95% CI: 4.5586 to 8.6236; $p < 0.0001$) (Figure 4A). No publication bias was found (t = 1.560; $p < 0.119$), nor was significant heterogeneity detected ($I^2 = 52.3883\%$, $p = 0.1331$) (Figure 4B).

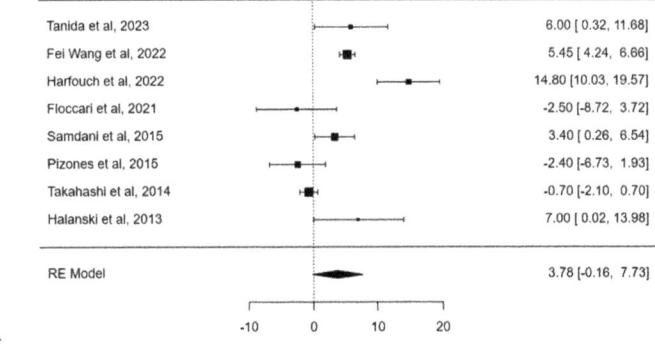

Figure 3. Cont.

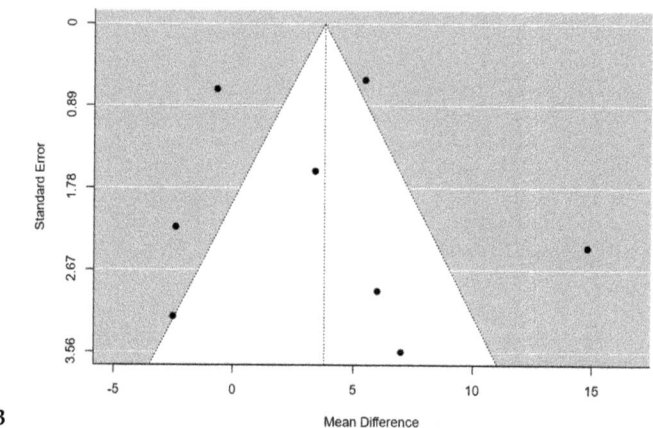

Figure 3. Forest plot (**A**) and funnel plot (**B**) of thoracic kyphosis change difference in meta-analysis between groups treated with and without POs [15–18,20–23].

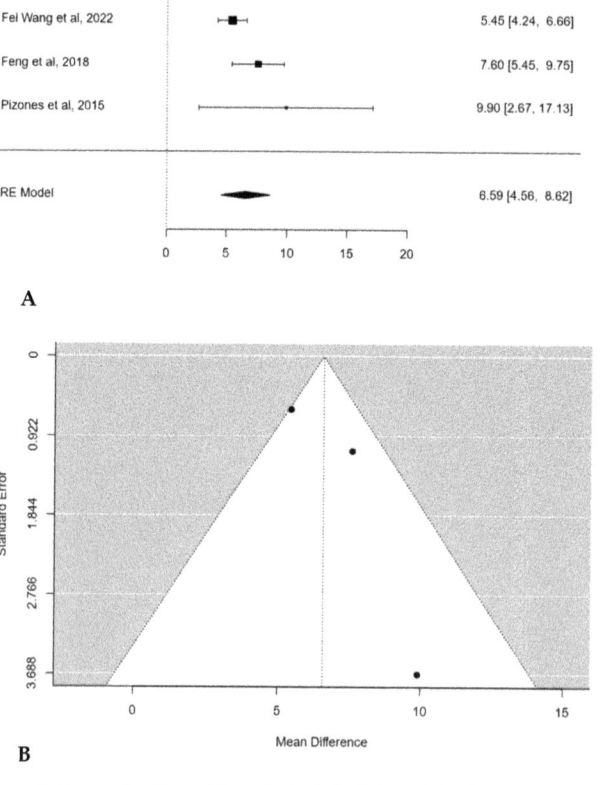

Figure 4. Forest plot (**A**) and funnel plot (**B**) of thoracic kyphosis change difference in meta-analysis between groups treated with and without POs, considering only hypokyphotic patients [17,19,23].

A further subgroup meta-analysis was performed in order to assess the mean TK change considering only normokyphotic patients (Lenke sagittal modifier N = 10° < TK < 40°). In this, three studies were included, and the estimated average mean TK change difference was

0.2° (95% CI: −5.9864 to 6.3258) without statistical significance ($p = 0.9569$) (Figure 5A). No publication bias was found (t = 0.121; $p < 0.903$), but significant heterogeneity was detected ($I^2 = 76.9945\%$, $p = 0.0114$) (Figure 5B).

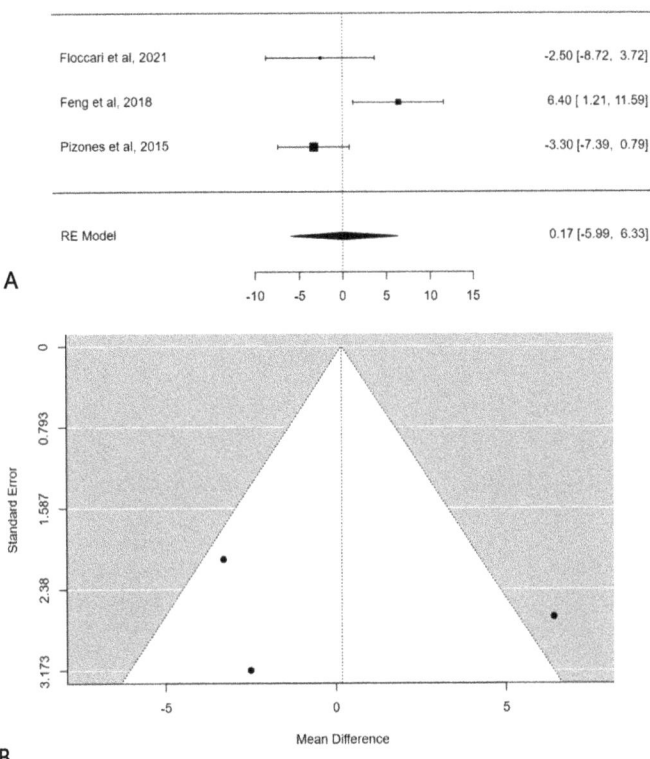

Figure 5. Forest plot (**A**) and funnel plot (**B**) of thoracic kyphosis change difference in meta-analysis between groups treated with and without POs, considering only normokyphotic patients [18,19,23].

3.3. Coronal Deformity Correction Rate

The mean Cobb angle of the major curve varied from 48.1 ± 3.9° [17] to 74.5 ± 15.2° [18], with a flexibility index ranging between 31.7% [21] and 54.5% [20]. Coronal correction rate of the major curve ranged between 62.0% [21] and 84.0% [15] in Pos groups, and from 58.7% [18] to 83.0% [15] in non-Pos groups.

Floccari et al. [18] reported the largest difference in the coronal correction rate of the major curve Cobb angle between Pos and non-Pos group, reporting 66.6% coronal correction with Pos and 58.7% without Pos ($p < 0.05$). No significant difference in coronal correction with and without Pos was found during the meta-analysis (2.5%; 95% CI: −0.5118 to 5.5179; $p = 0.1037$) (Figure 6A), despite most of the studies reported higher correction rates in patients who underwent PSF with POS [15,16,18,20,22]. Feng et al. [19] and Takahashi et al. [21] reported a higher correction rate in patients who underwent PSF without Pos. A significant publication bias (t = 4.65, $p < 0.001$) was found, and a moderate inconsistency among studies was found too ($I^2 = 82.7373\%$; $p < 0.0001$) (Figure 6B).

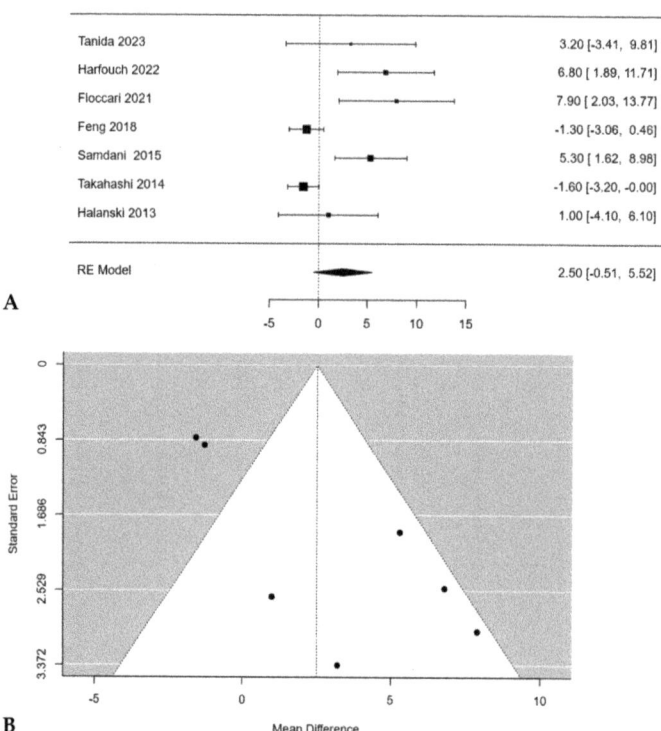

Figure 6. Forest plot (**A**) and funnel plot (**B**) of coronal correction rate difference in meta-analysis between groups treated with and without POs [15,16,18–22].

3.4. Surgical Time and Blood Loss

The mean surgical time ranged from 236.0 [21] to 368.2 [22] minutes with Pos, and from 187.0 [21] to 339.8 [22] minutes without Pos. Takahashi et al. [21], Feng et al. [19], and Fei Wang et al. [17] reported significantly higher surgical times in patients treated with POs ($p = 0.003$, $p < 0.001$ and $p < 0.001$, respectively).

A significant difference in surgical times between PSF with and without POs was found in the meta-analysis, with an estimated average mean difference of 21.5 min (95% CI: 0.5182 to 42.4744; $p = 0.0446$) (Figure 7A). Publication bias was found (t = -3.122, $p = 0.002$) and a substantial heterogeneity among studies was also revealed ($I^2 = 94.4656\%$, $p < 0.0001$) (Figure 7B).

The mean estimated blood loss (EBL) ranged from 619.7 [22] to 1141.0 mL [21] for patients treated with POs, and from 723.0 [22] to 979.8 mL [17] for patients treated without POs. Most authors reported significantly higher EBL in patients treated with POs [17,19–21], while Floccari et al. [18] and Tanida et al. [22] reported no significant differences in EBL between the two groups ($p = 0.825$ and $p = 0.28$, respectively).

Meta-analysis confirmed the statistical significance of estimated average mean EBL difference between PSF with and without Pos: 142.5 mL (95% CI: 1.7474 to 283.2643; $p = 0.0472$) (Figure 8A). No publication bias was found (t = -1.291, $p = 0.197$), but a substantial heterogeneity among studies was discovered ($I^2 = 91.7023\%$; $p < 0.0001$) (Figure 8B).

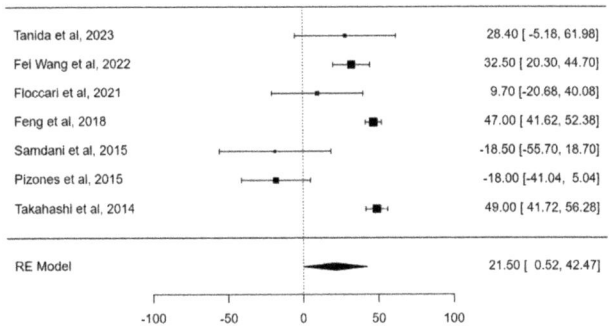

A

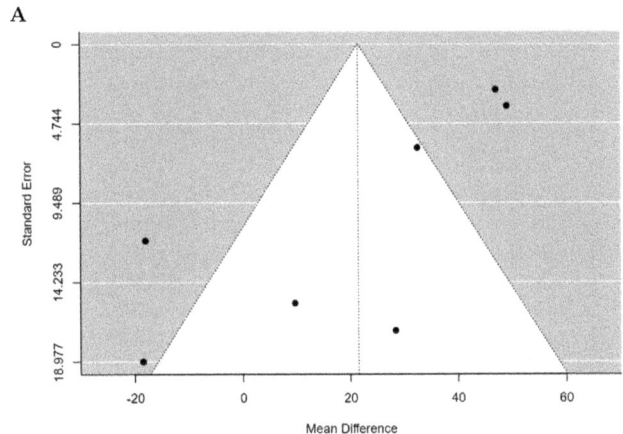

B

Figure 7. Forest plot (**A**) and funnel plot (**B**) of surgical time difference in meta-analysis between groups treated with and without POs [17–23].

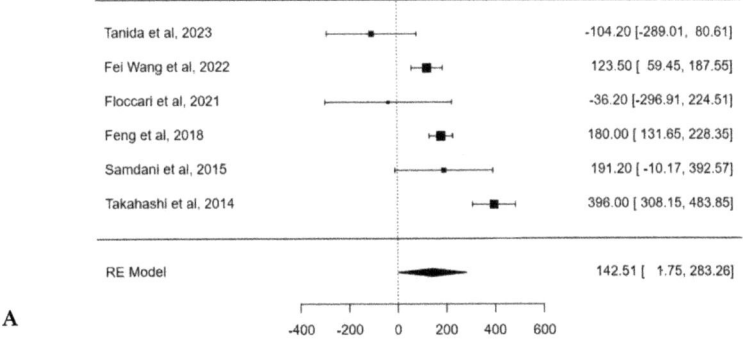

A

Figure 8. *Cont.*

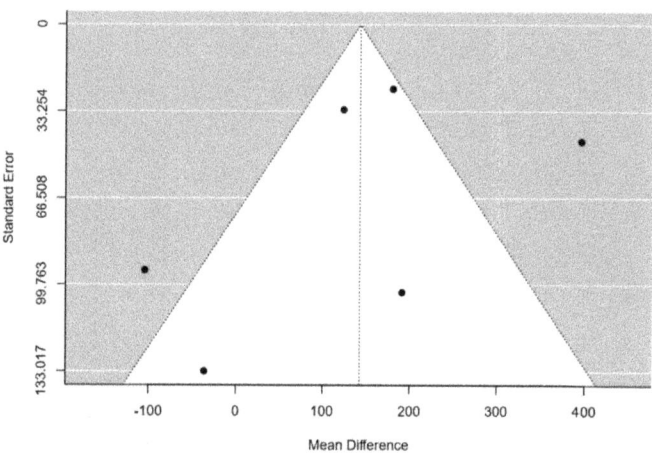

B

Figure 8. Forest plot (**A**) and funnel plot (**B**) of EBL difference in meta-analysis between groups treated with and without POs [17–22].

3.5. Complications

The complications rate ranged from 3.1 [19] to 34.2% [18] for patients treated with POs, and from 0 [16] to 6.1% [18] for patients treated without POs. Most authors reported higher complications rate in patients treated with POs [16–18], while Feng al. [19] and Halanski et al. [15] reported a similar complications rate between the two groups. Complications were reported and stratified according to the modified Clavien–Dindo–Sink classification [24] in Table 3.

Table 3. Reported complications stratified according to the modified Clavien–Dindo–Sink classification.

Author	Clavien–Dindo–Sink Grade I n (%) (Type)	Clavien–Dindo–Sink Grade II n (%) (Type)	Clavien–Dindo–Sink Grade III n (%) (Type)	Clavien–Dindo–Sink Grade I n (%) (Type)	Clavien–Dindo–Sink Grade IVb n (%) (Type)	Overall Complications n (%)
Fei Wang 2022 (P) [17]			2 (5%) (2 deep infections treated with surgical debridement and antibiotics)			2
Fei Wang 2022 (C) [17]			1 (2.5%) (1 case of abdominal pain treated with gastrointestinal decompression)			1 (2.5%)
Harfouch 2022 (P) [16]		3 (7.5%) (3 transient IONM changes that did not require staged surgery)	2 (5%) (2 IONM changes that required two-stage surgery with temporary rod)			5 (12.5%)
Harfouch 2022 (C) [16]						0
Floccari 2021 (P) [18]		4 (11.8%) (4 transient IONM changes that did not require staged surgery)	7 (20.6%) (1 IONM change that required two-stage surgery with temporary rod, 2 revisions for prominent implants, 1 revision for implant failure, 3 surgical debridements for surgical site infections)			11 (32.4%)

Table 3. Cont.

Author	Clavien–Dindo–Sink Grade I n (%) (Type)	Clavien–Dindo–Sink Grade II n (%) (Type)	Clavien–Dindo–Sink Grade III n (%) (Type)	Clavien–Dindo–Sink Grade I n (%) (Type)	Clavien–Dindo–Sink Grade IVb n (%) (Type)	Overall Complications n (%)
Floccari 2021 (C) [18]			2 (5.9) (1 reoperation for mechanical failure, 1 for infection)			2 (5.9%)
Feng 2018 (P) [19]	1 (3.1%) (1 hemopneumothorax treated with symptomatic and supportive treatments)					1 (3.1%)
Feng 2018 (C) [19]	2 (6.1%) (2 superficial surgical site infections treated with symptomatic and supportive treatments)					2 (6.1%)
Halanski 2013 (P) [15]	1 (5.9%) (pneumothorax)					1 (5.9%)
Halanski 2013 (C) [15]			1 (5.6%) (malpositioned screw that was removed)			1 (5.6%)

The meta-analysis reported an estimated average log odds ratio of 1.1 (95% CI: −0.1272 to 2.2511) with POs, which was not statistically significant ($p = 0.0801$) (Figure 9A). No publication bias (t = −0.200, $p = 0.817$) or substantial heterogeneity among studies was found ($I^2 = 22.1072\%$; $p = 0.3$) (Figure 9B).

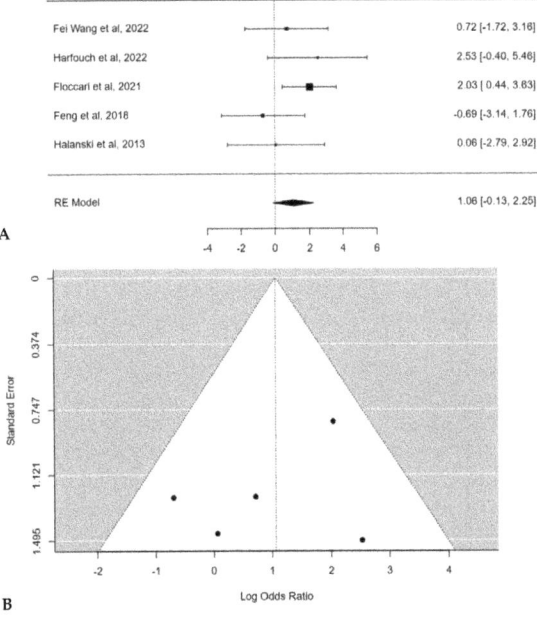

Figure 9. Forest plot (**A**) and funnel plot (**B**) of complications rate difference in meta-analysis between groups treated with and without POs [15–19].

4. Discussion

When considering all the eligible studies, the present work showed that the use of POs does not lead to a significant difference in TK change after AIS correction, with an estimated average mean difference of +3.8° (95% CI: −0.1644 to 7.7319°; $p = 0.0603$).

However, when performing a subgroup meta-analysis including only hypokyphotic patients, the use of POs led to a significantly greater TK increase (+6.6°; $p < 0.0001$). These results must be seen in light of some important considerations. In fact, POs should just be considered as release procedures that improve spinal flexibility, allowing for the surgeon to shape the desired final sagittal profile of the spine more efficiently. In that view, in hypokyphotic patients, POs may allow for a more efficient posterior translation of the spine to the over-contoured concave rod, reducing, on one side, the risk of rod deformation and, on the other side, reducing the risk of screws' pull-out. In addition to its statistical significance, it is crucial to determine if the difference in TK change achieved with the use of POs may also be clinically significant in hypokyphotic patients. In this regard, although slight when considered in absolute terms (+6.6°), the difference is actually remarkable when considered relative to the starting TK value (<10°), although we still do not know if this TK change may produce a true clinical difference. However, it must be noted that TK measurement can be challenging, particularly in AIS patients due to axial rotation and frontal inclination of vertebral bodies, with a reported measurement error of 6.68° (95% confidence interval 5.74–7.61°) [25]. In this view, apart from its unknown clinical significance, the estimated average TK increase of 6.6° may not overcome the measurement error.

An additional subgroup analysis was conducted considering only normokyphotic patients (TK between 10° and 40°), with an estimated average TK change difference of 0.2° (95% CI: −5.9864 to 6.3258; $p = 0.9569$). Although few studies were eligible, in this subset of patients, the use of POs did not seem to be supported by a better control of TK. In fact, interestingly, two studies [18,23] noticed a better TK control without POs. The possible explanation of this result is complex. In normokyphotic patients, the thoracic spine does not need a powerful posterior translation since TK is supposed to be physiologic. In these patients, TK should be preserved by a thoroughly performed corrective manoeuvre, alongside an accurate concave rod contouring. If DVR is inappropriately performed, exerting a pushing effect on the convex side, and if rods contouring is not adequate, a TK flattening may be seen. In this situation, the adoption of POs, due to their release effect, may even worsen the flattening effect generated by an incorrect deroto-translation.

Regarding the coronal correction rate, the use of POs did not lead a to a significant difference (2.5%; 95% CI: −0.5118 to 5.5179; $p = 0.1037$). However, it must be noted that the average coronal Cobb angle of the studies included in the analysis ranged between 50.8–74.5° and that the flexibility index ranged between 31.7 and 54.5%. Therefore, this result seems to apply only to non-severe, non-stiff, coronal deformities. Conversely, some authors [11,26] adopted multiple asymmetric POs for the management of severe (>90°) and stiff (flexibility index < 25%) curves. Unfortunately, these were not comparative studies, so they were not suitable for the present analysis. This may reflect an underlying selection bias, since surgeons who are comfortable with this kind of osteotomy would typically use them as an alternative to tricolumn-osteotomies when addressing severe and stiff curves in order to have a more powerful coronal translation and perform selective apical convex compression.

Regarding surgical time, the analysis showed a significantly longer operation time of 21.5 min (95% CI: 0.5182 to 42.4744; $p = 0.0446$) for POs groups. It is uncertain if such a mild difference in surgical time may be clinically significant, However, the fact that that many confounding factors could play a role must be considered (average fused levels, average implant density, average number of POs). Conversely, EBL was significantly greater in the POs groups (142.5 mL; 95% CI: 1.7474 to 283.2643; $p = 0.0472$). This result is not unexpected and it is in accordance with many previous studies [27,28]. Whether this difference in EBL may play a significant role in the clinical outcomes and in the risk of transfusion is still uncertain, especially considering that many factors can help reduce blood loss (tranexamic acid [29], ∈-aminocaproic acid [30], topical haemostatic agents [31]). Finally, we looked at the complications rate of POs. The meta-analysis reported an estimated average log odds ratio of 1.1 (95% CI: -0.1272 to 2.2511), which was not statistically significant ($p = 0.0801$). In addition to generic complications like mechanical failures or surgical site infections, which were represented in both groups, interestingly, two authors [16,18] reported 5 cases each of intraoperative neuromonitoring (IONM) changes in their POs groups. Many studies [32–34] related this specific complication to POs. This is difficult to interpret since many factors have an influence on IONM. On the metabolic side, the increased blood loss resulting from POs may lead to a spinal cord hypoperfusion and subsequent IONM change. On the mechanical side, the elongation of the posterior column in hypokyphotic patients, resulting from a distraction manoeuvre at the osteotomies sites, in addition to the elongation of the spine due to the correction of the coronal deformity, may overstretch the spinal cord.

The present study does not come without limitations. Firstly, many of the included studies did not have TK restoration as the main goal, which certainly may have led to a selection bias. Moreover, only a few studies performed a separate analysis of TK change in hypo-, normo- and hyperkyphotic patients. There is also a possible issue in the measurement method of TK since its measurement on plain X-rays can be extremely difficult in AIS patients, even when measured between T5 and T12. This in part due to an overshadowing effect by native thoracic anatomy and in part due the axial plane rotation of the vertebral bodies, which does not allow for a true lateral view with a 2d imaging [35,36]. This could be overcome by the adoption of 3D imaging TK measurement but, unfortunately, none of the included studies adopted such a measurement method. Moreover, the lack of 3D imaging analysis may underestimate the tridimensional corrective effect achieved with POs. This is exacerbated by the fact that it was not possible to conduct an axial plane meta-analysis, since only three studies reported axial plane corrections, with heterogeneous methods (two papers adopted scoliometer [18,20], one paper adopted CT scan [22]). Furthermore, the included studies were heterogeneous for what concerns baseline characteristics of the included patients. In particular, many studies comprised patients with different Lenke patterns: Harfouch et al. [16], Floccari et al. [18], Feng et al. [19], Pizones et al. [23], and Takahashi et al. [21] included double (III and VI) or triple curves (IV); meanwhile, all patients included by Tanida et al. [22], Fei Wang et al. [17], Samdani et al. [20], and Halanski et al. [15] had thoracic patterns (I or II). This may be a source of bias, since thoracic patterns tend to have less TK, while double and triple curves are more frequently normokyphotic. Moreover, only one study matched POs and non-POs cohorts; this may inevitably raise the variability between the patients in the POs and non-POs groups in each of the included studies. More crucially, many additional surgical factors with a possible influence on coronal and/or sagittal correction should have been more specially taken into account by the included studies. Specifically, pedicle screw density was specified just in two papers [18,21]; number of POs was specified by most [16–18,20–22] but not all authors [15,19,23]; rod material and diameter were not reported by two authors [19,20]. It should be further considered that the studies that reported rod material and diameter were highly heterogeneous in terms of their choices: some adopted 5.5 mm cobalt-chrome [16,17], some 6.35 stainless steel [23], and some hybrid choices (6 mm cobalt-chrome in concavity + 6 mm titanium alloy in convexity [22]). Moreover, some authors even adopted different rod choices among their cohorts of patients [15,18,21] and this may consequently account for some of the differences in the correction outcomes between POs and non-POs groups among these studies. Although screw density, number of Pos, and rod choice may be important factors in AIS surgical correction outcomes, they must be viewed as tools in the surgeon's hands. In fact, particularly regarding sagittal plane restoration, in a multicenter study by Monazzam et al. [37], the only significant predictor of TK restoration was the surgeon. This emphasizes the importance of the intraoperative corrective technique, especially in terms of rod contouring and regarding how and which corrective forces are applied by the surgeon. Despite that, many of the included papers did not provide an accurate technique description [15,18,21], and one paper was a multicenter study [20] with an inevitable heterogeneity in surgical technique.

Finally, all the included studies had a retrospective, non-randomized design, which may possibly represent an additional source of bias. Despite that, this is the first meta-analysis on the highly debated topic regarding TK control with the use of POs during AIS surgery, and the fact that only comparative studies were included helped to keep the internal variability of each study as low as possible. Further comparative studies, with better stratified patients according to preoperative TK and more precise measurement methods, will further shed a light on this topic.

5. Conclusions

Ponte osteotomies allow for significant restoration of TK in hypokyphotic AIS curves, without a significantly greater TK change in normokyphotic patients. On the coronal plane, a significantly greater correction rate was not reported, despite the included studies not focusing on severe and/or stiff curves. Considering the significantly greater EBL and the trend toward a higher complications rate, it appears clear that the correct indication of POs is crucial. Particularly in hypokyphotic patients, the benefits of TK restoration may overcome the risks. Conversely, the routinary use of POs in non-severe, non-stiff, and normokyphotic curves should be discouraged.

Author Contributions: Conceptualization, G.V. and C.F.; methodology, G.V. and M.T.; software, G.V. and M.T.; formal analysis, G.V. and M.T.; investigation, M.M., M.I., F.S., A.C. and S.C.P.; data curation, G.V. and M.T.; writing—original draft preparation, C.F., G.V. and M.T.; writing—review and editing, C.F., A.R., G.V. and M.T.; visualization, G.V. and M.T.; supervision, C.F. and A.R. All authors have read and agreed to the published version of the manuscript.

Funding: This research received no external funding.

Institutional Review Board Statement: Not applicable.

Informed Consent Statement: Not applicable.

Data Availability Statement: The data presented in this study are available in article.

Conflicts of Interest: The authors declare no conflict of interest.

References

1. Guo, X.; Chau, W.-W.; Chan, Y.-L.; Cheng, J.C.-Y. Relative anterior spinal overgrowth in adolescent idiopathic scoliosis. Results of disproportionate endochondral-membranous bone growth. *J. Bone Jt. Surg. Br.* **2003**, *85*, 1026–1031. [CrossRef] [PubMed]
2. Bodendorfer, B.M.; Shah, S.A.; Bastrom, T.P.; Lonner, B.S.; Yaszay, B.; Samdani, A.F.; Miyanji, F.; Cahill, P.J.; Sponseller, P.D.; Betz, R.R.; et al. Restoration of Thoracic Kyphosis in Adolescent Idiopathic Scoliosis Over a Twenty-year Period: Are We Getting Better? *Spine* **2020**, *45*, 1625–1633. [CrossRef]
3. Watanabe, K.; Nakamura, T.; Iwanami, A.; Hosogane, N.; Tsuji, T.; Ishii, K.; Nakamura, M.; Toyama, Y.; Chiba, K.; Matsumoto, M. Vertebral derotation in adolescent idiopathic scoliosis causes hypokyphosis of the thoracic spine. *BMC Musculoskelet. Disord.* **2012**, *13*, 99. [CrossRef] [PubMed]
4. Mladenov, K.V.; Vaeterlein, C.; Stuecker, R. Selective posterior thoracic fusion by means of direct vertebral derotation in adolescent idiopathic scoliosis: Effects on the sagittal alignment. *Eur. Spine J.* **2011**, *20*, 1114–1117. [CrossRef]
5. Di Silvestre, M.; Lolli, F.; Bakaloudis, G.; Maredi, E.; Vommaro, F.; Pastorelli, F. Apical vertebral derotation in the posterior treatment of adolescent idiopathic scoliosis: Myth or reality? *Eur. Spine J.* **2013**, *22*, 313–323. [CrossRef] [PubMed]
6. Kim, Y.J.; Lenke, L.G.; Kim, J.; Bridwell, K.H.; Cho, S.K.; Cheh, G.; Sides, B. Comparative analysis of pedicle screw versus hybrid instrumentation in posterior spinal fusion of adolescent idiopathic scoliosis. *Spine* **2006**, *31*, 291–298. [CrossRef] [PubMed]
7. Lowenstein, J.E.; Matsumoto, H.; Vitale, M.G.; Weidenbaum, M.; Gomez, J.A.; Lee, F.Y.-I.; Hyman, J.E.; Roye, D.P., Jr. Coronal and Sagittal Plane Correction in Adolescent Idiopathic Scoliosis: A comparison between all pedicle screw versus hybrid thoracic hook lumbar screw constructs. *Spine* **2007**, *32*, 448–452. [CrossRef]
8. Bernstein, P.; Hentschel, S.; Platzek, I.; Hühne, S.; Ettrich, U.; Hartmann, A.; Seifert, J. Thoracal flat back is a risk factor for lumbar disc degeneration after scoliosis surgery. *Spine J.* **2014**, *14*, 925–932. [CrossRef]

9. Hwang, S.W.; Samdani, A.F.; Tantorski, M.; Cahill, P.; Nydick, J.; Fine, A.; Betz, R.R.; Antonacci, M.D. Cervical sagittal plane decompensation after surgery for adolescent idiopathic scoliosis: An effect imparted by postoperative thoracic hypokyphosis. *J. Neurosurg. Spine* **2011**, *15*, 491–496. [CrossRef]
10. Demura, S.; Yaszay, B.; Carreau, J.H.; Upasani, V.V.; Bastrom, T.P.; Bartley, C.E.; Newton, P.O. Maintenance of Thoracic Kyphosis in the 3D Correction of Thoracic Adolescent Idiopathic Scoliosis Using Direct Vertebral Derotation. *Spine Deform.* **2013**, *1*, 46–50. [CrossRef]
11. Faldini, C.; Viroli, G.; Barile, F.; Manzetti, M.; Ialuna, M.; Traversari, M.; Vita, F.; Ruffilli, A. One stage correction via the Hi-PoAD technique for the management of severe, stiff, adolescent idiopathic scoliosis curves > 90°. *Spine Deform.* **2023**, *11*, 957–967. [CrossRef] [PubMed]
12. Ponte, A.; Orlando, G.; Siccardi, G.L. The True Ponte Osteotomy: By the One Who Developed It. *Spine Deform.* **2018**, *6*, 2–11. [CrossRef] [PubMed]
13. Moher, D.; Liberati, M.; Tetzlaff, J.; Altman, D.G.; PRISMA Group. Preferred reporting items for systematic reviews and meta-analyses: The PRISMA statement. *PLoS Med.* **2009**, *6*, e1000097. [CrossRef] [PubMed]
14. Sterne, J.A.C.; Hernán, M.A.; Reeves, B.C.; Savović, J.; Berkman, N.D.; Viswanathan, M.; Henry, D.; Altman, D.G.; Ansari, M.T.; Boutron, I.; et al. ROBINS-I: A tool for assessing risk of bias in non-randomised studies of interventions. *BMJ* **2016**, *355*, i4919. [CrossRef]
15. Halanski, M.A.; Cassidy, J.A. Do multilevel Ponte osteotomies in thoracic idiopathic scoliosis surgery improve curve correction and restore thoracic kyphosis? *J. Spinal Disord. Tech.* **2013**, *26*, 252–255. [CrossRef]
16. Harfouch, E.B.; Bunyan, R.F.; Al Faraidy, M.; Alnemari, H.H.; Bashir, S. Ponte osteotomies increase risk of intraoperative neuromonitoring alerts in adolescent idiopathic scoliosis surgery. *Surg. Neurol. Int.* **2022**, *13*, 154. [CrossRef] [PubMed]
17. Wang, F.; Chen, K.; Ji, T.; Ma, Y.; Huang, H.; Zhou, P.; Wei, X.; Chen, Z.; Bai, Y. Do hypokyphotic adolescent idiopathic scoliosis patients treated with Ponte osteotomy obtain a better clinical efficacy? A preliminary retrospective study. *J. Orthop. Surg. Res.* **2022**, *17*, 491. [CrossRef] [PubMed]
18. Floccari, L.V.; Poppino, K.; Greenhill, D.A.; Sucato, D.J. Ponte osteotomies in a matched series of large AIS curves increase surgical risk without improving outcomes. *Spine Deform.* **2021**, *9*, 1411–1418. [CrossRef]
19. Feng, J.; Zhou, J.; Huang, M.; Xia, P.; Liu, W. Clinical and radiological outcomes of the multilevel Ponte osteotomy with posterior selective segmental pedicle screw constructs to treat adolescent thoracic idiopathic scoliosis. *J. Orthop. Surg. Res.* **2018**, *13*, 305. [CrossRef]
20. Samdani, A.F.; Bennett, J.T.; Singla, A.R.; Marks, M.C.; Pahys, J.M.; Lonner, B.S.; Miyanji, F.; Shah, S.A.; Shufflebarger, H.L.; Newton, P.O.; et al. Do Ponte Osteotomies Enhance Correction in Adolescent Idiopathic Scoliosis? An Analysis of 191 Lenke 1A and 1B Curves. *Spine Deform.* **2015**, *3*, 483–488. [CrossRef]
21. Takahashi, J.; Ikegami, S.; Kuraishi, S.; Shimizu, M.; Futatsugi, T.; Kato, H. Skip pedicle screw fixation combined with Ponte osteotomy for adolescent idiopathic scoliosis. *Eur. Spine J.* **2014**, *23*, 2689–2695. [CrossRef] [PubMed]
22. Tanida, S.; Masamoto, K.; Tsukanaka, M.; Futami, T. No short-term clinical improvement and mean 6° of thoracic kyphosis correction using limited-level Ponte osteotomy near T7 for Lenke type 1 and 2 adolescent idiopathic scoliosis: A preliminary study. *J. Pediatr. Orthop. B* **2023**, *32*, 537–546. [CrossRef] [PubMed]
23. Pizones, J.; Sánchez-Mariscal, F.; Zúñiga, L.; Izquierdo, E. Ponte osteotomies to treat major thoracic adolescent idiopathic scoliosis curves allow more effective corrective maneuvers. *Eur. Spine J.* **2015**, *24*, 1540–1546. [CrossRef]
24. Dodwell, E.R.; Pathy, R.; Widmann, R.F.; Green, D.W.; Scher, D.M.; Blanco, J.S.; Doyle, S.M.; Daluiski, A.; Sink, E.L. Reliability of the Modified Clavien-Dindo-Sink Complication Classification System in Pediatric Orthopaedic Surgery. *JBJS Open Access* **2018**, *3*, e0020. [CrossRef] [PubMed]
25. Kuklo, T.R.; Potter, B.K.; Schroeder, T.M.; O'brien, M.F. Comparison of manual and digital measurements in adolescent idiopathic scoliosis. *Spine* **2006**, *31*, 1240–1246. [CrossRef]
26. Mirzashahi, B.; Moosavi, M.; Rostami, M. Outcome of Posterior-Only Approach for Severe Rigid Scoliosis: A Retrospective Report. *Int. J. Spine Surg.* **2020**, *14*, 232–238. [CrossRef] [PubMed]
27. Koerner, J.D.; Patel, A.; Zhao, C.; Schoenberg, C.B.; Mishra, A.; Vives, M.J.; Sabharwal, S. Blood loss during posterior spinal fusion for adolescent idiopathic scoliosis. *Spine* **2014**, *39*, 1479–1487. [CrossRef]
28. Dong, Y.; Tang, N.; Wang, S.; Zhang, J.; Zhao, H. Risk factors for blood transfusion in adolescent patients with scoliosis undergoing scoliosis surgery: A study of 722 cases in a single center. *BMC Musculoskelet. Disord.* **2021**, *22*, 13. [CrossRef] [PubMed]
29. Yoo, J.S.; Ahn, J.; Karmarkar, S.S.; Lamoutte, E.H.; Singh, K. The use of tranexamic acid in spine surgery. *Ann. Transl. Med.* **2019**, *7*, S172. [CrossRef] [PubMed]
30. Iorio, J.; Bennett, J.T.; Orlando, G.; Singla, A.; Dakwar, E.; Bonet, H.; Samdani, A.F. Does Amicar affect blood loss in patients with adolescent idiopathic scoliosis treated with pedicle screws and Ponte osteotomies? *Surg. Technol. Int.* **2013**, *23*, 291–295.
31. Baird, E.O.; McAnany, S.J.; Lu, Y.; Overley, S.C.; Qureshi, S.A. Hemostatic Agents in Spine Surgery: A Critical Analysis Review. *JBJS Rev.* **2015**, *3*. [CrossRef]
32. Lee, C.S.; Hwang, C.-J.; Lee, D.-H.; Cho, J.H.; Park, S. Risk Factors and Exit Strategy of Intraoperative Neurophysiological Monitoring Alert During Deformity Correction for Adolescent Idiopathic Scoliosis. *Glob. Spine J.* **2023**, 21925682231164344. [CrossRef] [PubMed]

33. Buckland, A.J.; Moon, J.Y.; Betz, R.R.; Lonner, B.S.; Newton, P.O.; Shufflebarger, H.L.; Errico, T.J.; Harms Study Group. Ponte Osteotomies Increase the Risk of Neuromonitoring Alerts in Adolescent Idiopathic Scoliosis Correction Surgery. *Spine* **2019**, *44*, E175–E180. [CrossRef] [PubMed]
34. Feng, B.; Qiu, G.; Shen, J.; Zhang, J.; Tian, Y.; Li, S.; Zhao, H.; Zhao, Y. Impact of multimodal intraoperative monitoring during surgery for spine deformity and potential risk factors for neurological monitoring changes. *J. Spinal Disord. Tech.* **2012**, *25*, E108–E114. [CrossRef]
35. Perdriolle, R.; Le Borgne, P.; Dansereau, J.; de Guise, J.; Labelle, H. Idiopathic scoliosis in three dimensions: A succession of two-dimensional deformities? *Spine* **2001**, *26*, 2719–2726. [CrossRef] [PubMed]
36. Parvaresh, K.C.; Osborn, E.J.; Reighard, F.G.; Doan, J.; Bastrom, T.P.; Newton, P.O. Predicting 3D Thoracic Kyphosis Using Traditional 2D Radiographic Measurements in Adolescent Idiopathic Scoliosis. *Spine Deform.* **2017**, *5*, 159–165. [CrossRef]
37. Monazzam, S.; Newton, P.O.; Bastrom, T.P.; Yaszay, B.; Harms Study Group. Multicenter Comparison of the Factors Important in Restoring Thoracic Kyphosis During Posterior Instrumentation for Adolescent Idiopathic Scoliosis. *Spine Deform.* **2013**, *1*, 359–364. [CrossRef]

Disclaimer/Publisher's Note: The statements, opinions and data contained in all publications are solely those of the individual author(s) and contributor(s) and not of MDPI and/or the editor(s). MDPI and/or the editor(s) disclaim responsibility for any injury to people or property resulting from any ideas, methods, instructions or products referred to in the content.

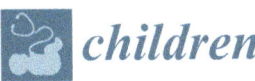

Article

Adolescent Idiopathic Scoliosis Surgery: Postoperative Functional Outcomes at 32 Years Mean Follow-Up

Giuseppe Barone [1], Fabrizio Giudici [1], Francesco Manzini [2], Pierluigi Pironti [2], Marco Viganò [3], Leone Minoia [1], Marino Archetti [1], Antonino Zagra [1] and Laura Scaramuzzo [1,*]

1. Spine Surgery Division 1, IRCCS Ospedale Galeazzi—Sant'Ambrogio, 20157 Milan, Italy; giuseppe.barone@grupposandonato.it (G.B.); fabrizio.giudici@grupposandonato.it (F.G.); leominoia@tin.it (L.M.); marino.archetti@grupposandonato.it (M.A.); laura.scaramuzzo@grupposandonato.it (A.Z.)
2. Residency Program in Orthopedics and Traumatology, University of Milan, 20122 Milan, Italy; francesco.manzini@unimi.it (F.M.)
3. IRCCS Ospedale Galeazzi—Sant'Ambrogio, 20157 Milan, Italy; marco.vigano@grupposandonato.it
* Correspondence: scaramuzzolaura@gmail.com

Abstract: Introduction: Recent clinical and radiographic studies conducted over short and medium terms have demonstrated positive results in patients undergoing surgery for adolescent idiopathic scoliosis (AIS). However, the absence of long-term data, crucial for comprehending the impact on future quality of life, especially in young patients actively involved in very intense physical activities, remains a gap. This study aims to evaluate long-term functional outcomes in patients who underwent surgery for Adolescent Idiopathic Scoliosis. Material and Methods: Patients meeting specific criteria (diagnosis of AIS, age at surgery between 12 and 18 years, and follow-up of at least 20 years) were identified from a large spine surgery center database. A questionnaire using "Google Form" assessed various outcomes, including Visual Analog Scale (VAS) back, VAS leg, Short Form 12 score (SF-12), Scoliosis Research Society 22 score (SRS-22), incidence of spine revision surgery, postoperative high demanding activities (work and sport), and possible pregnancies was sent to the enrolled patients. The authors analyzed the results regarding all patients included and, moreover, statistical analysis categorized patients into two groups based on the surgical fusion performed: Group 1 (non-instrumented technique according to Hibbs–Risser) and Group 2 (instrumented tecnique according to Cotrel–Dubousset). Results: A total of 63 patients (mean age 47.5 years) were included, with a mean follow-up of 31.9 years. Patients were, in mean, 47.5 years old. Group 1 comprised 42 patients, and Group 2 had 21 patients. Revision surgery was required in 19% of patients, predominantly for implant issues in Group 2 (11.9% vs. 33%, $p < 0.05$). Overall outcomes were favorable: VAS back = 3.5, VAS leg = 2.5, SRS-22 = 3.5, SF-12 Physical Component Summary = 41.1, SF-12 Mental Component Summary = 46.7, with no significant differences between the group 1 and group 2. At 5-years FU, the non-reoperation rate was higher in the non-instrumented group (97.6% vs. 71.4%, $p < 0.001$). By means of SRS-22, overall satisfaction was 3.7 ± 1.2 on a maximum scale of 5. More than half of women have successfully completed one pregnancy. Most patients (87.3%) maintained regular work activity. Among sport practioners, half returned to the similar preoperative level. Conclusions: This study reveals favorable long-term functional results in adolescent idiopathic scoliosis patients after surgical fusion. Mild to moderate back and leg pain were observed, but overall satisfaction, sport participation, and work activity were high. Surgical technique (non-instrumented vs. instrumented) did not significantly impact long-term results, though the instrumented fusion exhibited a higher revision rate.

Keywords: scoliosis; spine surgery; fusion; functional outcome

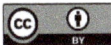

1. Introduction

The current literature suggest that adolescent idiopathic scoliosis has an estimated prevalence of 0.47–5.2% [1], using a cutoff point of 10° Cobb or more. AIS develops at the age of 10–18 years and the incidence for females is 1.4–2.1 times higher than for males. Survival analysis assessed that 0.7–1% of diagnosed patients underwent surgical treatment within five years. Surgery was most frequently performed at 12–14 years of age [2].

Whether or not an AIS patient should undergo surgical intervention depends on several factors including the overall curve size and pattern, curve progression, and skeletal maturity. Surgery is considered in skeletally immature patients with structural curve Cobb angles over 40° [3]. The natural evolution of adolescent idiopathic scoliosis (AIS) is unclear, especially for Cobb angles between 30° and 60° in adolescence. Historically, there is no clear consensus on the exact cutoff for scoliosis surgery, several factors including the overall size and pattern, curve progression, and skeletal maturity. In the recent past, a cutoff was set at 50° with a progressive reduction to 40° [3]. Otherwise, surgery is also recommended in immature patients with a progressive structural curve in the last six months of observation, in which important residual growth is expected.

Correction and fusion surgery have been used for the treatment of scoliosis since the early 1900. Russell Hibbs performed the first scoliosis fusion by posterior open release and uninstrumented "in situ" fusion with subsequent prolonged cast-immobilization from 6 to 12 months. Driven by the desire to increase the amount of deformity correction rate and to reduce the nonunion rate, surgical techniques including the use of internal instrumentation were investigated and developed over the years. Harrington rods (1960s), Luque sublaminar wires (1970s), laminar hooks, and pedicle screws by Cotrel and Dubusset (1970s, 1980s) have been used to present.

Today, patients can be treated with different surgical approaches: anterior spinal fusion, posterior spinal fusion, or a combined approach. It is estimated that currently 75% of AIS surgery is performed with a posterior-only approach [4]. New implants, new surgical approaches/techniques, and modern technology result in better surgical outcomes.

Since most of patients affected by scoliosis undergo surgery at a very young age, it is important to know long-term results, especially with regard to clinical outcomes and future quality of life. Many young patients carry out activities with high-functional demand, such as sports or work, and for this reason both patients and their parents are very interested to obtaining excellent long-term functional results. Today, in the literature there are mostly short- and medium-term follow-up. The purpose of this study is to evaluate the long-term functional outcomes in young patients who underwent surgery for adolescent idiopathis scoliosis, paying special attention to pain, social and sport activities, overall satisfaction, and quality of life. Another aim is to assess if the first instrumented fusion techniques lead to better long-term results than the older non-instrumented fusion technique and to find out possible differences in revision rate.

2. Materials and Methods

This retrospective cohort study was conducted at IRCCS Ospedale Galeazzi—Sant'Ambrogio, Milan (Italy), Spine Surgery Division 1.

A database of 509 patients who underwent surgical treatment for scoliosis by our spinal surgery division from 1980 to 2001 was analyzed. The database included the following information: patients' identity, diagnosis, age at surgery, other pathological conditions, date of surgery, detailed surgical procedure performed (extension of fusion, non-instrumented, or instrumented posterior technique).

We included patients diagnosed with AIS, age at surgery $\geq$ 12 and $\leq$18 years, undergoing posterior surgery, and with a follow-up greater than 20 years. Exclusion criteria were age at surgery > 18 years, other etiology (neurologic, syndromic, congenital).

After the first database review, 302 patients met the inclusion criteria and were selected to supply contact information (email or telephone number) using our hospital patient management software. Among them, 133 patients were contacted, and a questionnaire drafted in the form of a "Google Form" was mailed to patients along with an invitation to participate in the study, after a telephone conversation during which patient consent was collected. A total of 63 patients completed the form and were included in the study (Figure 1).

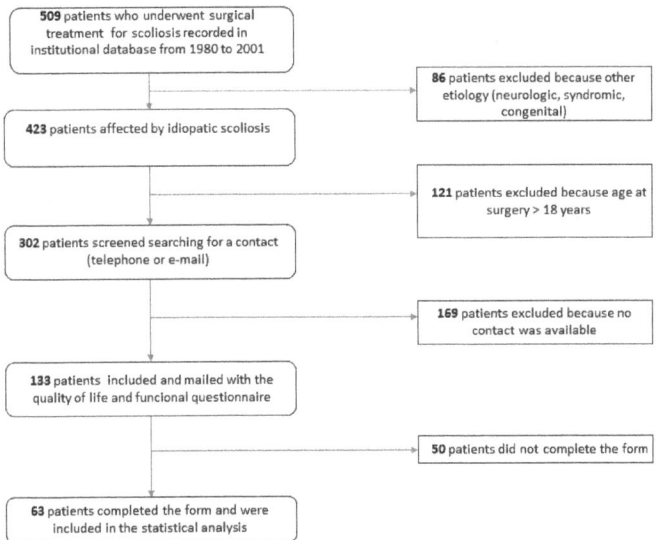

Figure 1. Flow diagram for inclusion and exclusion of patients in the study.

Through the questionnaire, we collected the following information: VAS back, VAS leg, Scoliosis Research Society 22 (SRS-22), Short Form 12 (SF-12), revision surgery rate, daily life aspects (pregnancy, work and sport activities).

Then, patients were further subdivided into two groups depending on the surgical procedure performed (Figure 2):

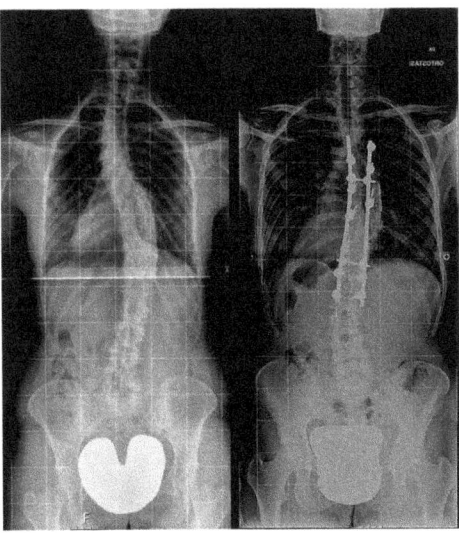

Figure 2. Examples of non-instrumented (**left**) and instrumented (**right**) long-term X-ray.

(1) Non-instrumented fusion according to Hibbs–Risser technique [5] (Group A): This technique is based on a meticulous fusion executed on each hemi-space, either on the concave side or the convex side of the curve.

The intervention, carried out following a median posterior surgical access, begins by identifying the supraspinous ligament, which is dissected longitudinally at the apex of the spinous apophysis and continuing to detach the periosteum from the two sides of the spinous process and, therefore, from the laminae, until reaching the transverse apophyses. Once the vertebral arches have been completely exposed and the capsular and ligamentous structures have been carefully eliminated, cortical bone is attacked by the chisel first removing the facet joints (inferior facet joint of the upper vertebra). In this way, a large quantity of autologous bone is obtained from the posterior structures (laminae, spinosa, transverse apophysis), which is prepared to obtain bone grafts that are reversed in sequence and applied at each level. In all cases, an iliac bone graft was applied to increase the fusion power.

The surgical treatment of scoliosis with the Risser technique involves preoperative correction (for a period of 3 months) and postoperative application of a cast (for a period of approximately 6 months).

(2) Instrumented posterior fusion according to Cotrel–Dubousset technique [6] (Group B): introduced in 1980s, this system uses double rods and multiple spinal posterior element fixation anchors. In our series, a hybrid construct involving lumbar pedicle screws and thoracic hooks was used. Pedicle screws were inserted using the freehand technique. All the instrumentations included a distal anchor by using four pedicle screws in the lower two vertebrae. Pedicle screws were applied in the lumbar spine and distal thoracic vertebrae (T9/T10). Instead, pedicle hooks were positioned in the proximal thoracic vertebrae with a cephalad direction. The hook was applied with the combination of a hook holder, a mallet, and a hook-pusher. In the convex side of the scoliotic curve, at the upper instrumented vertebra, a transverse process hook with a caudal direction was positioned to reach a stable anchor point. Screws at each level were applied alternatively on the concave and convex side of the scoliotic curve, but a greater density was usually performed on the concave side. The apical vertebra was always included in the instrumented vertebrae. The spinous process, supraspinous and interspinous ligament, and the other spine restraints were removed to facilitate the correction maneuvers. The laminae were fully and scrupulously decorticated. Bone graft obtained from decortication and bone removal was used for fusion, applying it directly to the posterior bone surfaces.

The scoliosis correction process began with the application of the first rod in the concave side of the main curve. The rods were previously accurately modeled to reproduce the correct sagittal shape of the instrumented spinal segment, paying attention to obtain the ideal thoracic kyphosis and lumbar lordosis. A balanced spine in the sagittal and coronal plane was a crucial goal to achieve; often, to prevent the remodeling of the prebent rods during correction, a hyper-kyphosis and hyper-lordosis were given when rods were modeled.

After bringing the rod closer to the screws, an initial correction was obtained by a segmental translation of the vertebrae toward the rod.

In practice, the rod was reduced into the reduction tabs to reach the screw head by using the setscrews.

Once the rods were engaged in all anchors, the surgeon and his assistant performed a global derotation of about 90° through the use of rod rotation instruments, in the direction of the concave side of the scoliotic curve, reaching the greatest degree of correction.

To obtain further correction and improve the deformity also on the axial plane, an additional segmental derotation was also performed.

When the patient was affected by a very stiff curve, additional correction maneuvers with segmental compression and distraction were applied [6].

For this study, we evaluated the functional outcomes of the entire cohort of patients and then divided them into the above groups and compared the results.

Statistical Analysis

The statistical analysis was performed using R Software v4.1.1 (R Core Team, Vienna, Austria). Continuous variables distribution was assessed by Shapiro–Wilk test. According to the result of this test, comparisons between groups were performed using Student t-test or Wilcoxon rank-sum test, in case of normal and non-normal distribution, respectively. Differences in the proportion of categorical variables were assessed by Fisher's exact test. p-Values < 0.05 were considered statistically significant.

3. Results

At the end of the inclusion and exclusion process, 63 patients respected inclusion criteria, sent the completed questionnaires, and were enrolled in the study for statistical analysis. Group A and B were, respectively, 42 and 21 patients. The mean age at surgery was 15.7 ± 1.8 years and the mean follow-up was 32 ± 7.3 years. When patients were interviewed via our questionnaire, the mean age was 47.5 ± 6.3 years. Mean age and follow-up among the two groups were different because the non-instrumented technique was older. The features of the patients are summarized in Table 1. The scoliotic curves were reevaluated from the radiographic images and were classified according to Lenke's classification (Lenke 1–21 patients; Lenke 3–18 patients; Lenke 5–18 patients; Lenke 6–4 patients; Lenke 3–2 patients). On average, 10.3 levels were fused, from a minimum of 8 to a maximum of 14 levels.

Table 1. Data about patients grouped in non-instrumented (Group A) and instrumented (Group B) techniques; differences between all patients, non-instrumented, and instrumented techniques groups; mean [standard deviation].

	All Patients	Group A Non-Instrumented	Group B Instrumented	p
Patients, n	63	42 (66.7%)	21 (33.3%)	-
Mean Age, year	47.5 ± 6.3	51.6 ± 5.1	37.3 ± 4.7	<0.001
Age at surgery, year	15.7 ± 1.8	15.6 ± 2	15.6 ± 2.1	0.538
F/M	57/6	39/13	18/3	0.391
Follow-up, year	32 ± 7.3	36.4 ± 3.9	23 ± 2.4	<0.001
Revision rate	12 (19%)	5 (11.9%)	7 (33%)	<0.05

Overall outcome measures (PROMs) showed good results in both groups, although 12 patients (19%) needed revision surgery, significantly more in the instrumented group (11.9% vs. 33%, $p < 0.05$).

The mean value of VAS back, VAS leg, Short Form 12 PCS, Short Form 12 MCS, and SRS-22 without group distinction resulted to be, respectively, 3.5 ± 3.11, 2.51 ± 2.7, 41.1 ± 11.8, 46.7 ± 9.8, and 3.5 ± 0.7. The average satisfaction score was 3.7 ± 1.2 out of a maximum value of 5. The groups comparison showed no significant differences in VAS back ($p = 0.533$), VAS leg ($p = 0.520$), SF-12 PCS ($p = 0.901$), SF-12 MCS ($p = 0.694$) as well as the SRS-22 ($p = 0.804$) (Figures 3 and 4).

The general satisfaction score was 3.7 ± 1.2 out of 5. The group comparison showed no statistically significant differences in VAS back ($p = 0.533$), VAS leg ($p = 0.520$), SF-12 PCS ($p = 0.901$), SF-12 MCS ($p = 0.694$) as well as the SRS-22 ($p = 0.804$) (Table 2).

Regarding survival rate, the two groups were significantly different (p-value < 0.001), with the greatest difference within the first 5 years. In fact, the rate of non-reoperation was 97.6% (CI95%: 84.3–100.0%) in the non-instrumented group and 71.4% (CI95%: 47.1–86.0%) in the instrumented group at 5-year follow-up (Figure 5).

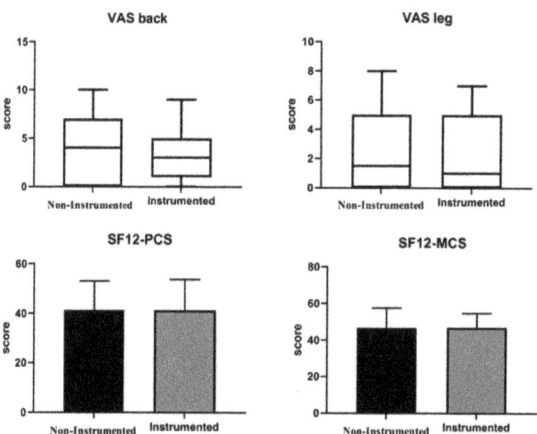

Figure 3. Functional outcomes reported by means of Tukey box and Whiskers plot with median (in-box line) and outliers (dots) in non-instrumented and instrumented fusions.

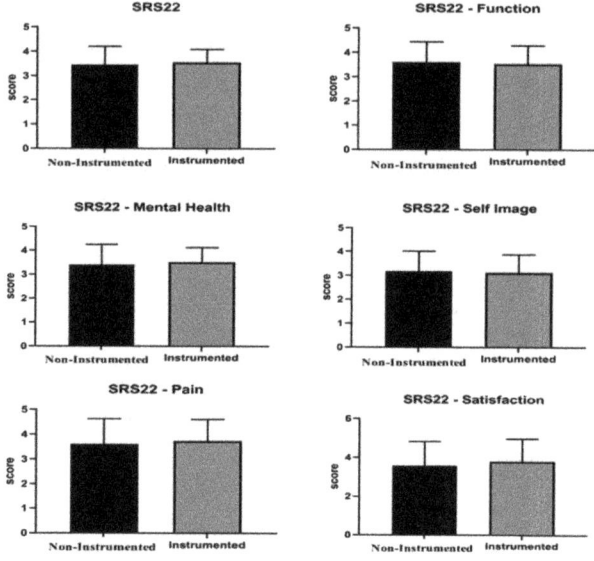

Figure 4. SRS22 general score and categories in non-instrumented and instrumented techniques.

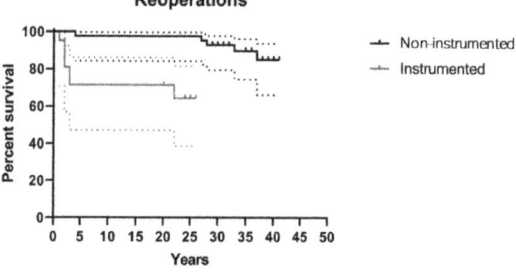

Figure 5. Survival curves depict the proportion of patients who did not undergo additional surgeries for each type of first intervention (non-instrumented and instrumented fusion).

Table 2. PROMs (patient-reported outcome measures) about patients grouped in non-instrumented (G1) and instrumented (G2) technique; differences between all patients, non-instrumented and instrumented technique groups; mean.

	All Patients	Non-Instrumented	Instumented	p
VAS back	3.5 ± 3.11	3.8 ± 3.3	3.1 ± 2.7	0.533
VAS leg	2.51 ± 2.7	2.7 ± 2.8	2.1 ± 2.7	0.520
SF-12 PCS	41.1 ± 11.8	41.3 ± 11.7	41.4 ± 12.3	0.901
SF-12 MCS	46.7 ± 9.8	46.7 ± 10.8	47 ± 7.8	0.694
SRS-22	3.5 ± 0.7	3.4 ± 0.7	3.5 ± 0.5	0.804
Function	3.6 ± 0.8	3.6 ± 0.8	3.5 ± 0.7	0.578
Pain	3.6 ± 0.9	3.6 ± 1	3.7 ± 0.9	0.703
Self Image	3.2 ± 0.8	3.2 ± 0.8	3.1 ± 0.8	0.994
Mental Health	3.4 ± 0.8	3.4 ± 0.8	3.5 ± 0.6	0.529
Satisfaction	3.7 ± 1.2	3.6 ± 1.2	3.8 ± 1.2	0.506

This was mainly due to implant issues.

Nevertheless, as stated before, a higher revision rate did not lead to worse long-term clinical results, as demonstrated by the comparable results between group A and group B in terms of pain, physical and mental state, and quality of life at long follow-up.

Overall, 87.3% of patients had stable jobs. The percentage was slightly lower in Group B than in Group A (85.7% vs. 88.1%). A successful pregnancy was achieved in 56% of all the patients: 59% in Group A and 50% in Group B (Table 3). A higher prevalence of cesarean sections compared to vaginal deliveries was assessed (21–65.6%–versus 11–34.4, respectively).

Table 3. Postoperative work activity and pregnancy.

Postoperative Work Activity and Pregnancy			
	ALL	NI-Technique	I-Techinque
Patients, n (%)	63	42 (66.7%)	21 (33.3%)
Work Activity–Stable job, n (%)	55 (87.3%)	37 (88.1%)	18 (85.7%)
Work Activity–Unemployed, n (%)	8 (12.7%)	8 (19%)	5 (23.8%)
All Female patients, n	57	39	18
Successful Pregnancy, n (%)	32 (56%)	23 (59%)	9 (50%)

A total of 34 patients (54% of the entire cohort) used to practice sport activities before surgery (50% amateur, 44.1% competitive, and 5.9% professional). A total of 79.4% of them returned to sport in the postoperative and 61.7% at last follow-up.

However, 20.6% (7 patients) stopped their sport because of thoracic and/or low back pain, functional limitation, or different reasons.

Dividing patients according to the level and intensity of sport activity, based on the American Academy of Pediatrics Classification [7], 47% of patients resumed a medium or high-intensity sport (level 3 or higher) in the postoperative, and 27% at last follow-up (Table 4).

Table 4. Level and intensity of sport activities, preoperatively, 1-year postoperative, and at the last follow-up.

	Preoperative	Postoperative	Last Follow-Up
All sports patients, n (%)	34	27 (79.4%)	21 (61.7%)
Level 1 (golf, bowling, walking)	/	/	5 (24%)
Level 2 (aerobic dancing, bicycling, jogging, swimming, tennis)	7 (21%)	14 (52%)	10 (48%)

Table 4. Cont.

	Preoperative	Postoperative	Last Follow-Up
Level 3 (fast running, weightlifting, high impact aerobic dancing, crew)	5 (17%)	5 (18.5%)	2 (9%)
Level 4 (gymnastic, volleyball, baseball, horseback riding, skating, skiing)	6 (18%)	3 (11%)	2 (9%)
Level 5 (basketball, boxing, football, soccer, martial arts, rugby)	16 (44%)	5 (18.5%)	2 (9%)
Amatorial	17 (50%)	18 (67%)	19 (91%)
Competitive	15 (44.1%)	8 (29%)	2 (9%)
Professional	2 (5.9%)	1 (4%)	0

4. Discussion

The present study shows a series of young patients operated for adolescent idiopathic scoliosis with long-term clinical follow-up. Our evaluation of the data does not intend to compare the results of two surgical techniques used for the treatment of AIS (non-instrumented and instrumented fusion). In fact, it would be useless to compare two techniques that are so different and developed several years apart. The main purpose of the study is to show the long-term clinical results of surgery especially on the quality of life of these young patients with high-functional demands. To our knowledge, this is one of the largest patients' series with such a long follow-up study of individuals surgically treated for AIS.

First, we confirmed the success and overall satisfaction of surgical treatment of scoliosis in patients with significant preoperative clinical alterations. The main indications for surgical treatment were AIS exceeding a certain degree of Cobb's angle (45°–50°), failure of conservative treatment, or symptomatic AIS [8], with still a wide range of differences according to the surgeon's preferences.

It should be noted that there is today no randomized or non-randomized trial-based evidence from prospective series with a control group comparing the outcomes of surgical to conservative treatments for patients affected by AIS and severe curves of over 45 degrees [9].

Akazawa et al. [10] compared 66 operated patients with 76 healthy age and sex-matched people with neither a history of spinal surgery nor spine deformity and found no statistical differences in back or leg pain, physical and mental health (SRS-22), and low back pain severity (RDQ) between patients and controls, indicating good long-term outcome of surgical treatment for AIS. Still, in Akazawa et al. function and self-image scores on the SRS-22 questionnaire were significantly lower in the AIS group than in the control group (function: 4.3 ± 0.6 and 4.7 ± 0.5 [$p < 0.0001$] and self-image: 3.0 ± 0.8 and 3.7 ± 0.5 [$p < 0.0001$], respectively). Another recent study by Farshad et al. [11] compared 16 operated patients with 16 matched patients with a conservatively treated AIS with a long-term follow-up (47 and 39 years, respectively, for the surgical and conservative group). They found no differences in functional scores (ODI score) but found a relevant smaller curve magnitude with surgical treatment (38° for surgery group vs 61° for conservative group at final follow-up, starting, respectively, from 48° and 40°). Ghandhari et al. [12], in a study on 42 patients and 5.6 years follow-up, found benefits about aesthetics, quality of life, disability, back pain, psychological well-being, and breathing function, but also alert about potential longer-term risks such as greater strain on unfused vertebrae, curvature progression, decompensation of the deformity, and degenerative disk disease.

The global functional results are still so good that, in the scientific literature, it is also confirmed that, after a spinal fusion for AIS, a full return to sport is generally allowed. Barile et al. [13], in their review of 2021, showed that a return to sport after surgery ranges from 6 to 18 months postoperatively, while operated patients can safely return to any sports. However, in some patients, especially after extremely long spine fusion, the loss of mobility could make it difficult for patients to play at the same level as preoperatively. According to Pepke et al. [14], 29.2% of a series of 33 patients operated of spinal fusion for AIS could return to the same level of preoperative sport activity. Many patients in this study who resumed sports postoperatively shifted from contact sports toward lower level and intensity sports activities. The extent of spinal fusion had no influence on the time to return to training and full sports-specific activity.

In our series, even many years after surgery, the maintenance of good clinical and functional scores for most of the patients is indicative of a high long-term satisfaction rate, improvement of clinical issues, and good overall quality of life. Despite the evidence of greater rate of surgical revision in instrumented group, good overall functional outcomes were found at last follow-up: SRS-22 = 3.5 ± 0.7, VAS back = 3.5 ± 3.11, VAS leg = 2.5 ± 2.7, SF-12 PCS = 41.1 ± 11.8, SF-12 MCS = 46.7 ± 9.8, indicating general good health, without statistical differences between two groups ($p > 0.05$) (Table 2).

With some surprise, our study demonstrates that even with the surgical technique that does not involve the use of instrumentation, the long-term functional outcomes are good and comparable to the most recent instrumented fusion technique. On the other hand, the higher rate of surgical revisions related to the use of implants in the instrumented fusion technique also does not appear to have a negative impact on long-term clinical follow-up in our series of patients.

In our series, the rate of non-reoperation was 97.6% (CI95%: 84.3–100.0%) in the non-instrumented group and 71.4% (CI95%: 47.1–86.0%) in the instrumented group at 5-year follow-up. The introduction of instrumentation increased the incidence of adverse event and need for revision, especially in the first years of use. In recent years, there has been also an increase in the need for revision in patients treated with the non-fusion technique. The need for revision is generally postponed till long-term follow-up in these patients of adult age, and it is linked to the progressive decompensation of the spine and degeneration of adjacent segment. However, as our results show, it does not always have an influence on clinical outcome.

General satisfaction score was 3.7 ± 1.2 out of a maximum value of 5; 56% of the women in our series had at least one successful pregnancy, and at the last follow-up 87% of the patients declared they were regularly employed. These data should help the surgeon to reassure parents and young patients during the decisional process about choosing the surgical treatment, a moment that could be very stressful for both [15]. Another good result is that, 32 years after surgery, only 20.6% of the operated patients declared to have stopped sport activity because of pain or other reasons, while 79.4% of them returned to sport in the postoperative and 61.7% at last follow-up.

The results of the present study are even more reassuring if we think that the surgical techniques have evolved considerably over the last two decades [16]. All screw instrumentations for posterior spine fusion are now performed in almost all cases (98.4%); major complication rates decreased over time (from 18.7% to 5.1% at two years follow-up); greater improvements were observed in satisfaction, back pain, function, and quality of life.

Our study has some limitations. First, it is a retrospective analysis and survey. The design of the study has potential recall bias. Even though the total number of patients is considerable if compared to other long-term studies in literature, the sample size is still quite small and does not allow a real statistical comparison between the two types of surgical techniques. However, as mentioned above, the primary objective is not to compare the results of two very different surgical techniques used for the treatment of AIS but to show the long-term clinical results of surgery especially on the quality of life of these young patients with high-functional demands. An important limitation of our series is the absence of radiographic findings; because of the difficulty in collecting pre- and postoperative radiographic images in patients surgically treated many years ago (with the risk of excluding further patients from the study), we preferred not to include the radiographic results in our outcomes, focusing only on functional results, which are more important for patient satisfaction.

5. Conclusions

Patients surgically treated for adolescent idiopathic scoliosis show good outcomes at long-term follow-up. Pain, function, physical and mental status, and overall satisfaction are good, both in non-instrumented and instrumented fusion techniques. Most patients resume high-level sport activity and carry out regular work activity. Despite the higher rate of surgical revision in the instrumented technique compared to the non-instrumented one, the long-term functional results are not significantly affected.

Author Contributions: G.B.: writing—original draft preparation; F.G.: methodology; F.M.: data curation; P.P.: data curation; M.V.: formal analysis, validation; L.M.: resources; M.A.: resources; A.Z.: project administration; L.S.: supervision, review and editing. All authors have read and agreed to the published version of the manuscript.

Funding: This research received no external funding.

Institutional Review Board Statement: The study was conducted in accordance with the Declaration of Helsinki. Ethical review and approval were waived for this study due to the retrospective nature of the study, and because it aims only to conduct a functional interview on treated patients without interference with their clinical follow-up.

Informed Consent Statement: Informed consent was obtained from all subjects involved in the study.

Data Availability Statement: Data will be available on Zenodo.org.

Acknowledgments: The APC was funded by Italian Ministry of Health—"Ricerca Corrente".

Conflicts of Interest: The authors declare no conflicts of interest.

References

1. Konieczny, M.R.; Senyurt, H.; Krauspe, R. Epidemiology of adolescent idiopathic scoliosis. *J. Child. Orthop.* **2013**, *7*, 3–9. [CrossRef] [PubMed]
2. Sung, S.; Chae, H.-W.; Lee, H.S.; Kim, S.; Kwon, J.-W.; Lee, S.-B.; Moon, S.-H.; Lee, H.-M.; Lee, B.H. Incidence and Surgery Rate of Idiopathic Scoliosis: A Nationwide Database Study. *Int. J. Environ. Res. Public Health* **2021**, *18*, 8152. [CrossRef] [PubMed]
3. Hopf, C. Criteria for treatment of idiopathic scoliosis between 40 degrees and 50 degrees. Surgical vs. conservative therapy. *Orthopade* **2000**, *29*, 500–506. [CrossRef] [PubMed]
4. Von Heideken, J.; Iversen, M.D.; Gerdhem, P. Rapidly increasing incidence in scoliosis surgery over 14 years in a nationwide sample. *Eur. Spine J.* **2018**, *27*, 286–292. [CrossRef] [PubMed]
5. Hibbs, R.A.; Risser, J.C.; Ferguson, A.B. Scoliosis treated by the fusion operation: An end-result study of three hundred and sixty cases. *J. Bone Jt. Surg.* **1931**, *13*, 91–104.
6. Cundy, P.; Paterson, D.; Hillier, T.; Sutherland, A.; Stephen, J.; Foster, B. Cotrel-Dubousset instrumentation and vertebral rotation in adolescent idiopathic scoliosis. *J. Bone Jt. Surg. Br.* **1990**, *72*, 670–674. [CrossRef] [PubMed]
7. American Academy of Pediatrics. Medical conditions affecting sports participation. *Pediatrics* **2001**, *107*, 1205–1209. [CrossRef] [PubMed]
8. Dolan, L.; Weinstein, S. Surgical rates after observation and bracing for adolescent idiopathic scoliosis: An evidence-based review. *Spine* **2007**, *32*, S91–S100. [CrossRef] [PubMed]
9. Bettany-Saltikov, J.; Weiss, H.-R.; Chockalingam, N.; Taranu, R.; Srinivas, S.; Hogg, J.; Whittaker, V.; Kalyan, R.V.; Arnell, T. Surgical versus non-surgical interventions in people with adolescent idiopathic scoliosis. *Cochrane Database Syst. Rev.* **2015**, CD010663. [CrossRef] [PubMed]
10. Akazawa, T.; Minami, S.; Kotani, T.; Nemoto, T.; Koshi, T.; Takahashi, K. Long-Term Clinical Outcomes of Surgery for Adolescent Idiopathic Scoliosis 21 to 41 Years Later. *Spine* **2012**, *37*, 402–405. [CrossRef] [PubMed]
11. Farshad, M.; Kutschke, L.; Laux, C.J.; Kabelitz, M.; Schüpbach, R.; Böni, T.; Jentzsch, T. Extreme long-term outcome of operatively versus conservatively treated patients with adolescent idiopathic scoliosis. *Eur. Spine J.* **2020**, *29*, 2084–2090. [CrossRef] [PubMed]
12. Ghandhari, H.; Ameri, E.; Nikouei, F.; Bozorgi, M.H.A.; Majdi, S.; Salehpour, M. Long-term outcome of posterior spinal fusion for the correction of adolescent idiopathic scoliosis. *Scoliosis Spinal Disord.* **2018**, *13*, 14. [CrossRef] [PubMed]
13. Barile, F.; Ruffilli, A.; Manzetti, M.; Fiore, M.; Panciera, A.; Viroli, G.; Faldini, C. Resumption of sport after spinal fusion for adolescent idiopathic scoliosis: A review of the current literature. *Spine Deform.* **2021**, *9*, 1247–1251. [CrossRef] [PubMed]
14. Pepke, W.; Madathinakam, A.; Bruckner, T.; Renkawitz, T.; Hemmer, S.; Akbar, M. Return to Sport after Adolescent Idiopathic Scoliosis (AIS) Correction Surgery: A Retrospective Data Analysis. *J. Clin. Med.* **2023**, *12*, 1551. [CrossRef] [PubMed]

15. Rullander, A.-C.; Isberg, S.; Karling, M.; Jonsson, H.; Lindh, V. Adolescents' Experience with Scoliosis Surgery: A Qualitative Study. *Pain Manag. Nurs.* **2013**, *14*, 50–59. [CrossRef] [PubMed]
16. Lonner, B.S.; Ren, Y.; Yaszay, B.; Cahill, P.J.; Shah, S.A.; Betz, R.R.; Samdani, A.F.; Shufflebarger, H.L.; Newton, P.O. Evolution of Surgery for Adolescent Idiopathic Scoliosis Over 20 Years: Have Outcomes Improved? *Spine* **2018**, *43*, 402–410. [CrossRef] [PubMed]

Disclaimer/Publisher's Note: The statements, opinions and data contained in all publications are solely those of the individual author(s) and contributor(s) and not of MDPI and/or the editor(s). MDPI and/or the editor(s) disclaim responsibility for any injury to people or property resulting from any ideas, methods, instructions or products referred to in the content.

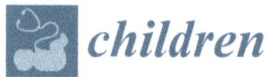

Article

Rod Angulation Relationship with Thoracic Kyphosis after Adolescent Idiopathic Scoliosis Posterior Instrumentation

Louis Boissiere [1,*], Anouar Bourghli [2], Fernando Guevara-Villazon [1], Ferran Pellisé [3], Ahmet Alanay [4], Frank Kleinstück [5], Javier Pizones [6], Cécile Roscop [7], Daniel Larrieu [1] and Ibrahim Obeid [1] on behalf of the European Spine Study Group

[1] ELSAN, Polyclinique Jean Villar, 53 Avenue Maryse Bastié, 33520 Bruges, France
[2] Spine Surgery Department, King Faisal Specialist Hospital and Research Center, Riyadh 11211, Saudi Arabia
[3] Spine Surgery Unit, Hospital Universitario Val Hebron, 08035 Barcelona, Spain
[4] Department of Orthopaedics and Traumatology, Acibadem University School of Medicine, Istanbul 34750, Turkey
[5] Research and Development, Schulthess Klinik, 8008 Zurich, Switzerland
[6] Spine Surgery Unit, Hospital Universitario La Paz, 28046 Madrid, Spain
[7] Spine Surgery Unit, CHU Pellegrin, 33076 Bordeaux, France
* Correspondence: dr.boissiere@cliniques-terrefort.fr

Abstract: Introduction: Surgery to correct spinal deformities in scoliosis involves the use of contoured rods to reshape the spine and correct its curvatures. It is crucial to bend these rods appropriately to achieve the best possible correction. However, there is limited research on how the rod bending process relates to spinal shape in adolescent idiopathic scoliosis surgery. Methods: A retrospective study was conducted using a prospective multicenter scoliosis database. This study included adolescent idiopathic scoliosis patients from the database who underwent surgery with posterior instrumentation covering the T4 to T12 segments. Standing global spine X-rays were used in the analysis. The sagittal Cobb angles between T5 and T11 were measured on the spine. Additionally, the curvature of the rods between T5 and T11 was measured using the tangent method. To assess the relationship between these measurements, the difference between the dorsal kyphosis (TK) and the rod kyphosis (RK) was calculated ($\Delta K = TK - RK$). This study aimed to analyze the correlation between ΔK and various patient characteristics. Both descriptive and statistical analyses were performed to achieve this goal. Results: This study encompassed a cohort of 99 patients, resulting in a total of 198 ΔK measurements for analysis. A linear regression analysis was conducted, revealing a statistically significant positive correlation between the kyphosis of the rods and that of the spine ($r = 0.77$, $p = 0.0001$). On average, the disparity between spinal and rod kyphosis averaged 5.5°. However, it is noteworthy that despite this modest mean difference, there was considerable variability among the patients. In particular, in 84% of cases, the concave rod exhibited less kyphosis than the spine, whereas the convex rod displayed greater kyphosis than the spine in 64% of cases. It was determined that the primary factor contributing to the flattening of the left rod was the magnitude of the coronal Cobb angle, both before and after the surgical procedure. These findings emphasize the importance of considering individual patient characteristics when performing rod bending procedures, aiming to achieve the most favorable outcomes in corrective surgery. Conclusions: Although there is a notable and consistent correlation between the curvature of the spine and the curvature of the rods, it is important to acknowledge the substantial heterogeneity observed in this study. This heterogeneity suggests that individual patient factors play a significant role in shaping the outcome of spinal corrective surgery. Furthermore, this study highlights that more severe spinal curvatures in the frontal plane have an adverse impact on the shape of the rods in the sagittal plane. In other words, when the scoliosis curve is more pronounced in the frontal plane, it tends to influence the way the rods are shaped in the sagittal plane. This underscores the complexity of spinal deformities and the need for a tailored approach in surgical interventions to account for these variations among patients.

Citation: Boissiere, L.; Bourghli, A.; Guevara-Villazon, F.; Pellisé, F.; Alanay, A.; Kleinstück, F.; Pizones, J.; Roscop, C.; Larrieu, D.; Obeid, I., on behalf of the European Spine Study Group. Rod Angulation Relationship with Thoracic Kyphosis after Adolescent Idiopathic Scoliosis Posterior Instrumentation. *Children* 2024, 11, 29. https://doi.org/10.3390/children11010029

Academic Editor: Reinald Brunner

Received: 10 October 2023
Revised: 30 November 2023
Accepted: 19 December 2023
Published: 26 December 2023

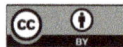

Copyright: © 2023 by the authors. Licensee MDPI, Basel, Switzerland. This article is an open access article distributed under the terms and conditions of the Creative Commons Attribution (CC BY) license (https://creativecommons.org/licenses/by/4.0/).

Keywords: adolescent idiopathic scoliosis; rod contour; thoracic kyphosis; predictive medicine; surgical planning

1. Introduction

The surgical management of adolescent idiopathic scoliosis (AIS) has evolved over the years, and the posterior approach instrumentation, correction, and fusion have emerged as the gold standard for treating this condition [1]. The success of this surgical procedure hinges on several key factors that play a crucial role throughout the operation. These factors include carefully selecting the appropriate fusion levels, achieving optimal rod bending in the sagittal plane, and executing precise reduction maneuvers [2].

The correction of the frontal plane deformity, which can be assessed by the measurement of the Cobb angle, has been a well-established part of scoliosis surgery for many years [3]. However, achieving sagittal plane correction is more challenging, especially when instrumentation of the thoracic spine is necessary [4]. One of the concerns during surgery is the potential for increasing thoracic kyphosis, which can impact the patient's overall spinal alignment [5].

Scoliosis typically leads to the flattening of the spine in most cases [6,7], emphasizing the importance of achieving a harmonious balance in the instrumented portion of the spine. To ensure the best possible outcome, meticulous preoperative surgical planning is indispensable [8]. This planning process helps formulate the surgical strategy and establish radiological goals, providing guidance for the surgical team [9].

The success of scoliosis surgery depends on various factors, and achieving optimal rod bending is among the critical elements [10]. Previous research has explored the intricate connection between proper rod bending and the successful execution of surgical planning [11]. Additionally, numerous studies have delved into the correlation between rod curvature and spinal curvature, employing diverse measurement methods. These investigations have encompassed degenerative spine surgery [12], spine trauma [13], adult spinal deformity (ASD) surgery [14], and AIS surgery [15]. However, it is noteworthy that the relationship between rod and spine curvatures may exhibit variations among these studies.

In recent times, there has been a growing interest in the development of specialized custom-made rods to achieve ideal corrections [11]. These rods are custom manufactured based on preoperative planning and are expected to offer superior correction compared to traditional rods manually bent by the surgeon during the procedure [16]. However, it is essential to underscore that the benefits of these specialized rods remain unproven, and there is currently no definitive data supporting the notion that these ideal rods consistently produce the best correction. It is crucial to recognize that various factors come into play during surgery, including compression and distraction maneuvers and the inherent flexibility of the spine.

During reduction maneuvers, the rod undergoes mechanical stress, leading to gradual deformation. This deformation results in a different shape for the rod before and after reduction, with some studies reporting an average angular loss of 20 degrees during AIS surgery, particularly in the concave portion of the curve [17]. To mitigate the risk of rod deformation, the choice of rod material (titanium alloy or cobalt chrome) or rod diameter (5.5 to 6 mm) can also influence deformation. As of now, there is no conclusive evidence favoring one type of rod over another [18]. Most studies report equivalent outcomes in terms of correction percentage, consolidation, or breakage, irrespective of the rod type used.

Given the complexity of the factors involved, there is still a vast field of investigation to fully comprehend the precise impact of reduction maneuvers. This raises the critical question of the predictability of surgical outcomes. A multitude of studies will be required to address these complex issues comprehensively [19].

However, as an initial step, the purpose of this study is to assess the relationship between rod shape and spinal shape on the first postoperative radiography. The primary inquiry revolves around whether the final shape of the rod can independently predict the ultimate shape of the spine in the thoracic fused spine after AIS surgery. Additionally, we aim to identify any predictive factors that may influence this relationship.

2. Material and Methods

2.1. Design

This study adopted a retrospective design, making use of a prospective multicenter database that centered its focus on operated adolescents for scoliosis and Scheuermann disease. The database's inclusion criteria encompassed individuals who had undergone surgery for AIS and Scheuermann kyphosis, all of whom were below 18 years old at the time of the initial assessment. Notably, the database did not include cases of congenital scoliosis.

From this extensive database, the study population consisted of patients who had undergone posterior fusion surgery for AIS. These patients were required to have a minimum follow-up period of 3 months, with their first postoperative X-ray serving as the baseline assessment. To maintain consistency and homogeneity in the study group, cases involving left thoracic major curves and Scheuermann kyphosis were excluded. The analysis focused on cases involving the fixation of spinal segments from T5 to T11.

In all instances, the upper instrumented vertebra (UIV) was positioned at T4 or higher, while the lower instrumented vertebra (LIV) was situated at T12 or lower. At the time of data extraction, the database included records for a total of 171 patients, of whom 72 patients were excluded from the subsequent analysis. Ultimately, this study included and analyzed data from 99 patients who met the specified criteria.

2.2. Surgery Technique

The surgical procedures were performed by multiple surgeons from four different spine centers, all following established standards for correcting adolescent idiopathic scoliosis. Notably, there were variations in the reduction techniques used across these centers. In all cases, posterior spinal pedicle screw instrumentation was utilized. To ensure surgical precision, neurophysiological monitoring was consistently applied throughout the procedures. The placement of pedicle screws was carried out using a combination of the freehand technique, fluoroscopy, or navigation, depending on the specific surgical site and timing.

In situations where the spine exhibited rigidity, posterior column osteotomies were conducted to enhance flexibility. Surgeons took into account the resulting thoracic kyphosis and lumbar lordosis when shaping the rods. To achieve the desired reduction, derotation and/or translation maneuvers were applied to one or both rods. In certain cases, additional in situ adjustments, such as over or under-contouring, along with interpedicular "compression-distraction" techniques, were employed to optimize the final construct.

This approach allowed for a comprehensive understanding of the surgical procedures performed across different centers while highlighting the variability in reduction techniques and the emphasis on precision throughout. It also underscored the importance of considering spine flexibility and adopting various maneuvers to achieve the desired correction during AIS surgery [6,20].

2.3. Data Collection and Radiographic Measurement

We collected demographic and radiographical data for our study. Radiographic analysis was performed using KEOPS® software (www.keops-spine.fr) based in Paris, France. The measurement of thoracic kyphosis (TK) in the T5-T11 region was conducted using the Cobb method, which determines the angle between the line parallel to the upper endplate of T5 and the line parallel to the lower endplate of T11 [21].

Additionally, we measured left and right rod kyphosis (RK) in the T5–T11 segment using the tangent method. This measurement involved calculating the angle formed by the perpendicular line to the tangent of the rod at the T5 and T11 screw positions [14] (Figure 1). To assess the difference between TK and RK, we computed the value ΔK, which is obtained by subtracting RK from TK ($\Delta K = TK - RK$). The gathered parameters are typically those regularly collected for assessing an AIS cohort, including age, gender, instrumented levels, rod specifications, and the primary Cobb angle measurement.

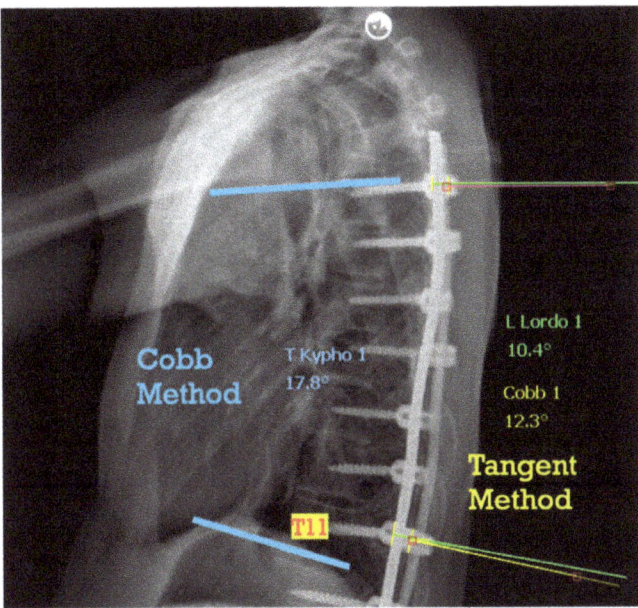

Figure 1. T5–T11 thoracic measurement with the Cob method and T5–T11 rod measurement with the tangent method.

2.4. Statistical Analysis

We summarized the descriptive parameters of the population using means and standard deviations. To assess the relationship between T5–T11 thoracic kyphosis (TK) and rod kyphosis (RK), we employed Pearson's correlation coefficient. Additionally, we graphed and measured the ΔK values. To investigate the associations between ΔK and other variables (preoperative and postoperative major Cobb angle, right and left rod), we conducted univariate analyses and calculated Pearson's correlation coefficients. Statistical significance was determined if the "p" value was less than 0.05. All statistical analyses were conducted using IBM SPSS Statistics 23.0 (SPSS Inc., Chicago, IL, USA).

3. Results

We analyzed a total of 198 rods from 99 patients. Table 1 summarizes the demographic data (gender, age), surgical details (instrumented levels, implants, osteotomies), and radiographic measurements (Cobb angle, kyphosis, lordosis, rod curvature, and ΔK).

The mean SRS-22 score significantly improved from 3.69 (SD 0.67) in preoperative to 4.29 (SD 0.73) in postoperative.

The average correction of the major curve in the coronal plane amounted to 42.4%, reducing from an initial measurement of 62.6° (SD 12.8) to 26.6° (SD 9.4). In contrast, the T5-T11 thoracic kyphosis exhibited a flattening trend, decreasing from 25.1° (SD 16.4) to 23.7° (SD 8.6). However, upon conducting a paired sample T-test, this change was found to be statistically non-significant ($p = 0.25$). It is important to note that this study did not distinguish between hypokyphotic and hyperkyphotic thoracic curves.

Table 1. Demographic and radiologic descriptive data.

Variable	Mean (Standard Deviation)	Cases
Gender		86 F, 13 M
Age	14 (1.6)	
Posterior Instrumented Levels	11 (2.6)	
Number of Implants	17 (5.1)	
Posterior Column Osteotomy		15 (14.1%)
Preoperative Major Cobb Angle	62.6° (12.8)	
Postoperative Major Cobb Angle	26.6° (9.4)	
Preoperative T5–T11 Kyphosis	25.1° (16.4)	
Postoperative T5–T11 Kyphosis	23.7° (8.6)	
Mean Rod Curvature (T5–T11)	20.9° (8.9)	
Preoperative Lumbar Lordosis	59.4° (23.1)	
Postoperative Lumbar Lordosis	58.3° (10.4)	
T5–T11 ΔK	2.7° (6)	
Mean Absolute T5–T11 ΔK	5.5° (3.6)	

The average measurement for thoracic kyphosis (TK) between T5 and T11 was 23.7° (SD 8.6), while the corresponding measurement for rod kyphosis (RK) was 20.9° (SD 8.9). A paired sample correlation analysis between T5-T11 RK and TK revealed consistent correlation values (R = 0.77, $p < 0.01$) (Figure 2).

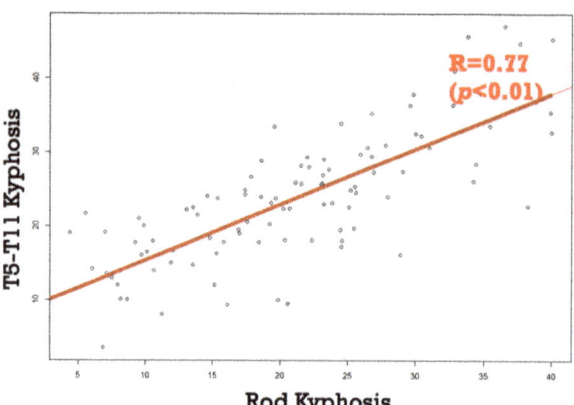

Figure 2. Strong correlation between rod and spine thoracic kyphosis.

The difference between TK and RK amounted to an average of 8.10° (SD 5.84). Notably, 75% of the values exhibited higher TK than RK, indicating a positive ΔK. Furthermore, 63% of the patients displayed a difference, in absolute value, of ΔK greater than 5° (Figure 3).

We conducted a comparison between the left rod, typically the concave rod, and the right convex rod. Our findings revealed that 84% of the left rods exhibited less kyphosis than thoracic kyphosis of the spine. Conversely, in the case of the right rods, 64% displayed greater kyphosis than the spine's thoracic kyphosis. Importantly, no significant differences in kyphosis were observed between the two rod materials, cobalt chrome and titanium alloy (Figure 4).

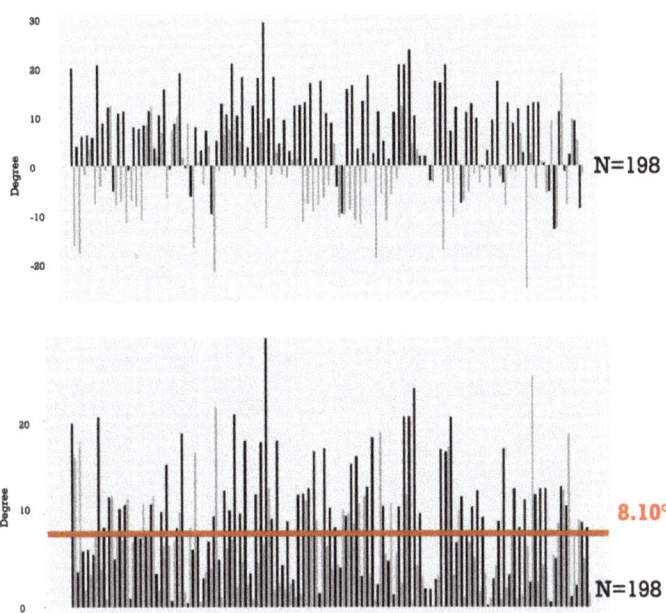

Figure 3. Numeric and absolute value of the difference between rod and spine kyphosis. The left rods are represented in black, while the right rods are shown in gray. The red line represents the mean average between the rod and spine kyphosis.

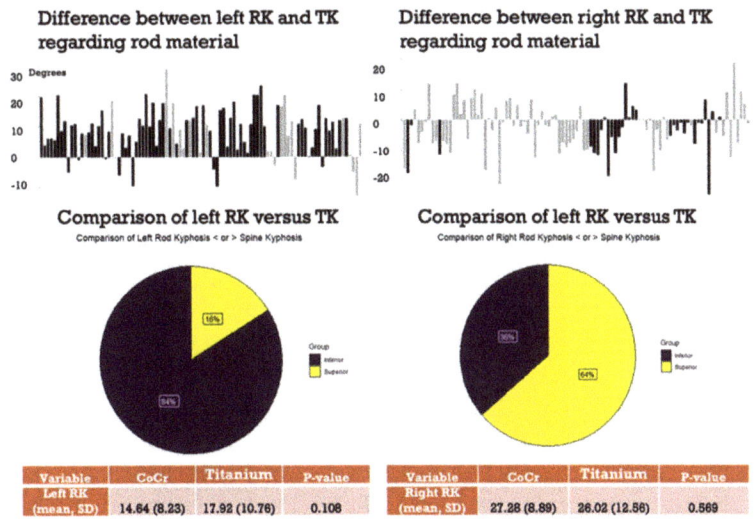

Figure 4. Differences between left and right rod and TK.

Both preoperative and postoperative thoracic kyphosis (TK) exhibited a strong correlation with the kyphosis of the left and right rods. In particular, a larger preoperative or postoperative Cobb angle was associated with a flatter left rod (correlation coefficients: r = 0.29 and r = 0.27, respectively). This correlation remained consistently strong when comparing the difference between preoperative and postoperative T5–T11 TK with the mean rod kyphosis (left and right) or the individual left and right rod kyphosis (Figure 5).

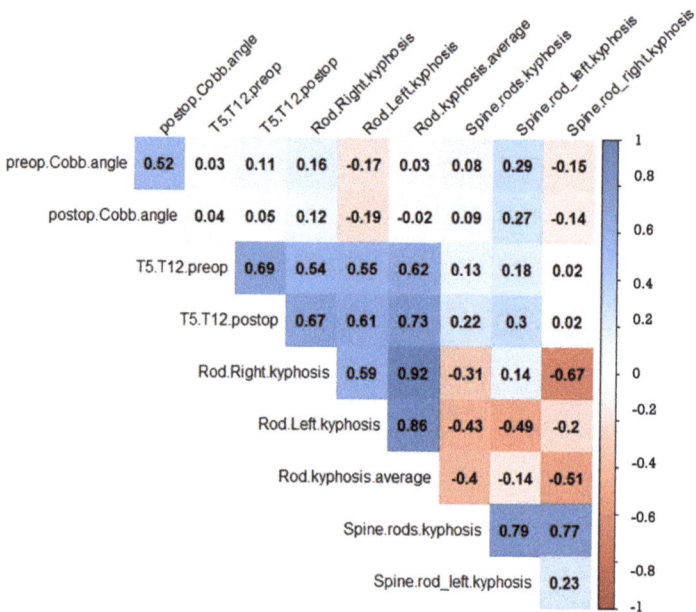

Figure 5. Significant correlation factors between preoperative, postoperative coronal Cobb angle, T5–T11 TK, and left and right RK. The blank squares are non-significant correlation factors.

4. Discussion

Despite the dearth of studies exploring the factors influencing surgical predictability, this study affirms a robust linear correlation between rod curvature and spine curvature. This underscores the critical role of proper rod bending in achieving desired postoperative results [22]. The sagittal plane restoration in spinal deformity surgery presents an intriguing challenge due to the inherent curvatures of the spine. The introduction of the Lenke classification brought sagittal plane analysis in AIS to the forefront and encouraged the adoption of various surgical techniques aimed at improving thoracic kyphosis [23–25]. The exact relationship between the rod and spine curvatures remains unclear. This study supports the fact that bending the rod will impact the final shape of the spine.

However, it is crucial to note that more than half of the rods deviated by over 5° from the expected thoracic kyphosis. This deviation raises valid questions about the rod's ability to reliably predict the final correction. The difference observed between concave and convex rods serves as a stark reminder that scoliosis is a three-dimensional deformity. Both rods play distinct roles in the reduction process, and their bending is influenced by both the desired final spinal shape and the mechanical stresses encountered during reduction maneuvers [26,27].

While AIS surgery employs very stiff rods, concave left rods have a propensity to flatten significantly. To counteract this effect, surgeons often recommend overbending the concave rod before commencing the reduction process [17]. Interestingly, our study did not reveal significant differences between titanium and cobalt chrome rods, implying that rod material may not exert a substantial influence on surgical outcomes. This observation aligns with existing literature that generally does not find material-dependent differences [28].

The parameter most closely correlated with rod flattening is the major Cobb angle in the coronal plane. A larger Cobb angle typically signifies a stiffer spine and a more substantial correction. However, much like previous studies, we encountered challenges in directly comparing the loss of kyphosis in rods before and after placement. Nevertheless, we concur that increasing the curvature of the concave rod remains essential. Nevertheless, the substantial variability observed between rod curvature and thoracic kyphosis suggests that relying solely on rod centering may be insufficient. Instead, the shape and rigidity of the spine are likely pivotal in determining the final rod shape.

In our study, the T5–T11 segment exhibited less kyphosis postoperatively compared to preoperative measurements. It is worth noting that our analysis intentionally focused on a specific spinal segment. We aimed to evaluate the relationship between rod and spine curvature more directly, rather than quantifying changes in kyphosis between pre- and postoperative states, a common approach in evaluating T4–T12 or T2–T12 kyphosis. The reason is to concentrate our attention on the completely fused part of the spine so that the results cannot be influenced by the adjacent mobile junctional segments.

As with any study, ours has several limitations. It is inherently retrospective and involves a variety of surgical strategies and techniques. Importantly, our study does not seek to evaluate the surgical outcomes of AIS correction; instead, its primary focus is on understanding the intricate relationship between the rod and spine curvature. Additionally, we must acknowledge the inherent complexity of scoliosis, a three-dimensional deformity being analyzed through two-dimensional parameters. This complexity necessitates further investigations aimed at refining predictive factors for final radiological outcomes. Beyond angular correction, elements such as transitional zones [29], apex location, and curve magnitude all warrant in-depth exploration to advance our understanding of AIS surgical correction.

5. Conclusions

For AIS correction surgery, the objective is often to increase thoracic kyphosis. The rod must be contoured appropriately and is strongly correlated with the spine's shape. Despite this correlation, in many cases, we observe significant variability between the curvature of the spine and the curvature of the rod. Multiple factors can explain this variability, but the anatomical factors linked to scoliosis itself (major Cobb angle) seem to be more impactful than surgical factors such as rod material. With these observations, it currently appears challenging to believe that a so-called 'ideal' rod would lead to a better correction.

Author Contributions: Conceptualization, L.B., F.G.-V. and I.O.; methodology, L.B., F.G.-V., I.O. and D.L.; software, D.L. and C.R.; validation, A.A, F.P., J.P., I.O. and F.K., formal analysis, D.L.; investigation, D.L.; resources, I.O., A.A., F.P., J.P. and F.K.; data curation, D.L.; writing L.B. and A.B.—original draft preparation, L.B.; writing—review and editing, L.B.; visualization, L.B.; supervision, L.B. and I.O.; project administration, L.B. and I.O.; funding acquisition, ESSG. All authors have read and agreed to the published version of the manuscript.

Funding: This research is funded by the European Spine Study Group.

Institutional Review Board Statement: The study was conducted in accordance with the Declaration of Helsinki, and approved by the Institutional Review Board of ELSAN (IRB#2023-10-OBEID-1 accessed on 26 October 2023).

Informed Consent Statement: Written informed consent has been obtained from the patient(s) to enter the ESSG registry and to use the data for clinical research purposes.

Data Availability Statement: The data presented in this study are available on request from the corresponding author. The data are not publicly available due to all data are part of the ESSG registry.

Conflicts of Interest: L.B.: Consultant Spineart, Spinevision; A.B.: no conflicts of interest; F.G.-V.; no conflicts of interest; F.P.: Research support: DePuySpine Synthes/Medtronic/Nuvasive/Orthofix/SpineArt, Consultant: Medtronic/Nuvasive; A.A.: Consultant: Globus, Zimvie, Research Grant: Depuy, Medtronic, Royalty: Zimvie; F.K.: Depuy Spine Speakers Bureau and Research Grant; J.P.: Consultant: Medtronic, Grants: medtronic Depuy; C.R.: consultant: clariance, spineart; D.L.: reserch support Medtronic, depuy; I.O.: consultant: Medtronic, spinevision, depuy; royalties: spinerat, clariance, alphatec, research support depuy, Medtronic.

References

1. Chen, Z.; Rong, L. Comparison of combined anterior–posterior approach versus posterior-only approach in treating adolescent idiopathic scoliosis: A meta-analysis. *Eur. Spine J.* **2016**, *25*, 363–371. [CrossRef] [PubMed]
2. Berlin, C.; Tielemann, S.; Quante, M.; Halm, H. Correlation of radiographic parameters and patient satisfaction in adolescent idiopathic scoliosis treated with posterior screw-dual-rod instrumentation. *Eur. Spine J.* **2023**, *32*, 3140–3148. [CrossRef] [PubMed]
3. King, H.A.; Moe, J.H.; Bradford, D.S.; Winter, R.B. The selection of fusion levels in thoracic idiopathic scoliosis. *J. Bone Jt. Surg. Am.* **1983**, *65*, 1302–1313. [CrossRef]
4. Bao, H.; Shu, S.; Yan, P.; Liu, S.; Liu, Z.; Zhu, Z.; Qian, B.; Qiu, Y. Fifteen Years and 2530 Patients: The Evolution of Instrumentation, Surgical Strategies, and Outcomes in Adolescent Idiopathic Scoliosis in a Single Institution. *World Neurosurg.* **2018**, *120*, e24–e32. [CrossRef] [PubMed]
5. Pesenti, S.; Clément, J.-L.; Ilharreborde, B.; Morin, C.; Charles, Y.P.; Parent, H.F.; Violas, P.; Szadkowski, M.; Boissière, L.; Jouve, J.-L.; et al. Comparison of four correction techniques for posterior spinal fusion in adolescent idiopathic scoliosis. *Eur. Spine J.* **2022**, *31*, 1028–1035. [CrossRef] [PubMed]
6. Pesenti, S.; Charles, Y.P.; Prost, S.; Solla, F.; Blondel, B.; Ilharreborde, B.; on behalf of the French Spine Surgery Society (SFCR). Spinal Sagittal Alignment Changes during Childhood: Results of a National Cohort Analysis of 1,059 Healthy Children. *J. Bone Jt. Surg.* **2023**, *105*, 676–686. [CrossRef] [PubMed]
7. Clément, J.-L.; Geoffray, A.; Yagoubi, F.; Chau, E.; Solla, F.; Oborocianu, I.; Rampal, V. Relationship between thoracic hypokyphosis, lumbar lordosis and sagittal pelvic parameters in adolescent idiopathic scoliosis. *Eur. Spine J.* **2013**, *22*, 2414–2420. [CrossRef]
8. Thomas, E.S.; Boyer, N.; Meyers, A.; Aziz, H.; Aminian, A. Restoration of thoracic kyphosis in adolescent idiopathic scoliosis with patient-specific rods: Did the preoperative plan match postoperative sagittal alignment? *Eur. Spine J.* **2023**, *32*, 190–201. [CrossRef]
9. Schlager, B.; Großkinsky, M.; Ruf, M.; Wiedenhöfer, B.; Akbar, M.; Wilke, H.-J. Range of surgical strategies for individual adolescent idiopathic scoliosis cases: Evaluation of a multi-centre survey. *Spine Deform.* **2023**. Ahead of print. [CrossRef]
10. Aubin, C.-E.; Labelle, H.; Ciolofan, O.C. Variability of spinal instrumentation configurations in adolescent idiopathic scoliosis. *Eur. Spine J.* **2007**, *16*, 57–64. [CrossRef]
11. Solla, F.; Barrey, C.Y.; Burger, E.; Kleck, C.J.; Fière, V. Patient-specific Rods for Surgical Correction of Sagittal Imbalance in Adults: Technical Aspects and Preliminary Results. *Clin. Spine Surg. Spine Publ.* **2019**, *32*, 80–86. [CrossRef] [PubMed]
12. Moufid, A.Y.; Cloche, T.; Ghailane, S.; Ounajim, A.; Vendeuvre, T.; Gille, O. Mismatch between rod bending and actual post-operative lordosis in lumbar arthrodesis with poly axial screws. *Orthop. Traumatol. Surg. Res.* **2019**, *105*, 1143–1148. [CrossRef] [PubMed]
13. Shi, Z.; Wang, G.; Jin, Z.; Wu, T.; Wang, H.; Sun, J.; Nicolas, Y.S.M.; Rupesh, K.C.; Yang, K.; Liu, J. Use of the sagittal Cobb* angle to guide the rod bending in the treatment of thoracolumbar fractures: A retrospective clinical study. *J. Orthop. Surg. Res.* **2020**, *15*, 574. [CrossRef] [PubMed]
14. Boissiere, L.; Guevara-villazón, F.; Bourghli, A.; Abdallah, R.; Pellise, F.; Pizones, J.; Alanay, A.; Kleinstueck, F.; Larrieu, D.; Obeid, I. Rod angulation does not reflect sagittal curvature in adult spinal deformity surgery: Comparison of lumbar lordosis and rod contouring. *Eur. Spine J.* **2023**, *32*, 3666–3672. [CrossRef] [PubMed]
15. Wang, X.; Boyer, L.; Le Naveaux, F.; Schwend, R.M.; Aubin, C.-E. How does differential rod contouring contribute to 3-dimensional correction and affect the bone-screw forces in adolescent idiopathic scoliosis instrumentation? *Clin. Biomech.* **2016**, *39*, 115–121. [CrossRef]
16. Solla, F.; Barrey, C.Y.; Rampal, V.; Fière, V. Comments to "Utility of Patient-Specific Rod Instrumentation in Deformity Correction: Single Institution Experience" by Sadrameli et al. *Spine Surg. Relat. Res.* **2021**, *5*, 450–451. [CrossRef]
17. Le Navéaux, F.; Aubin, C.-E.; Parent, S.; Newton, P.O.; Labelle, H. 3D rod shape changes in adolescent idiopathic scoliosis instrumentation: How much does it impact correction? *Eur. Spine J.* **2017**, *26*, 1676–1683. [CrossRef]
18. Sabah, Y.; Clément, J.-L.; Solla, F.; Rosello, O.; Rampal, V. Cobalt-chrome and titanium alloy rods provide similar coronal and sagittal correction in adolescent idiopathic scoliosis. *Orthop. Traumatol. Surg. Res.* **2018**, *104*, 1073–1077. [CrossRef]
19. Pasha, S.; Shah, S.; Newton, P. Machine Learning Predicts the 3D Outcomes of Adolescent Idiopathic Scoliosis Surgery Using Patient–Surgeon Specific Parameters. *Spine* **2021**, *46*, 579–587. [CrossRef]
20. Terai, H.; Toyoda, H.; Suzuki, A.; Dozono, S.; Yasuda, H.; Tamai, K.; Nakamura, H. A new corrective technique for adolescent idiopathic scoliosis: Convex manipulation using 6.35 mm diameter pure titanium rod followed by concave fixation using 6.35 mm diameter titanium alloy. *Scoliosis* **2015**, *10*, S14. [CrossRef]
21. McAlister, W.H.; Shackelford, G.D. Measurement of spinal curvatures. *Radiol. Clin. N. Am.* **1975**, *13*, 113–121. [CrossRef] [PubMed]
22. Burke, C.A.; Speirs, J.N.; Nelson, S.C. Maximizing mechanical advantage: Surgical technique increases stiffness in spinal instrumentation. *Spine Deform.* **2022**, *10*, 295–299. [CrossRef] [PubMed]
23. Clement, J.-L.; Chau, E.; Kimkpe, C.; Vallade, M.-J. Restoration of Thoracic Kyphosis by Posterior Instrumentation in Adolescent Idiopathic Scoliosis: Comparative Radiographic Analysis of Two Methods of Reduction. *Spine* **2008**, *33*, 1579–1587. [CrossRef] [PubMed]
24. Lenke, L.G.; Betz, R.R.; Harms, J.; Bridwell, K.H.; Clements, D.H.; Lowe, T.G.; Blanke, K. Adolescent idiopathic scoliosis: A new classification to determine extent of spinal arthrodesis. *J. Bone Jt. Surg. Am.* **2001**, *83*, 1169–1181. [CrossRef]

25. Pesenti, S.; Lafage, R.; Henry, B.; Kim, H.J.; Bolzinger, M.; Elysée, J.; Cunningham, M.; Choufani, E.; Lafage, V.; Blanco, J.; et al. Deformity correction in thoracic adolescent idiopathic scoliosis: A comparison of posteromedial translation using sublaminar bands and cantilever with pedicle screws. *Bone Jt. J.* **2020**, *102-B*, 376–382. [CrossRef] [PubMed]
26. Kluck, D.; Newton, P.O.; Sullivan, T.B.; Yaszay, B.; Jeffords, M.; Bastrom, T.P.; Bartley, C.E. A 3D Parameter Can Guide Concave Rod Contour for the Correction of Hypokyphosis in Adolescent Idiopathic Scoliosis. *Spine* **2020**, *45*, E1264–E1271. [CrossRef] [PubMed]
27. Wan, S.H.-T.; Wong, D.L.-L.; To, S.C.-H.; Meng, N.; Zhang, T.; Cheung, J.P.-Y. Patient and surgical predictors of 3D correction in posterior spinal fusion: A systematic review. *Eur. Spine J.* **2023**, *32*, 1927–1946. [CrossRef]
28. Ilharreborde, B.; Simon, A.L.; Ferrero, E.; Mazda, K. How to Optimize Axial Correction without Altering Thoracic Sagittal Alignment in Hybrid Constructs with Sublaminar Bands: Description of the "Frame" Technique. *Spine Deform.* **2019**, *7*, 245–253. [CrossRef]
29. Stagnara, P.; Claude De Mauroy, J.; Dran, G.; Gonon, G.P.; Costanzo, G.; Dimnet, J.; Pasquet, A. Reciprocal Angulation of Vertebral Bodies in a Sagittal Plane: Approach to References for the Evaluation of Kyphosis and Lordosis. *Spine* **1982**, *7*, 335–342. [CrossRef]

Disclaimer/Publisher's Note: The statements, opinions and data contained in all publications are solely those of the individual author(s) and contributor(s) and not of MDPI and/or the editor(s). MDPI and/or the editor(s) disclaim responsibility for any injury to people or property resulting from any ideas, methods, instructions or products referred to in the content.

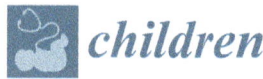

Review

Minimally Invasive Surgery for Posterior Spinal Instrumentation and Fusion in Adolescent Idiopathic Scoliosis: Current Status and Future Application

Ludmilla Bazin [1,†], Alexandre Ansorge [2,†], Tanguy Vendeuvre [3], Blaise Cochard [1], Anne Tabard-Fougère [1,*], Oscar Vazquez [1], Giacomo De Marco [1], Vishal Sarwahi [4] and Romain Dayer [1]

1. Division of Paediatric Orthopaedics, Faculty of Medicine, Geneva University Hospitals, 1211 Geneva, Switzerland; oscar.vazquez@hcuge.ch (O.V.)
2. Department of Spine Surgery, Lucerne Cantonal Hospital, 6000 Lucerne, Switzerland
3. Department of Orthopedic and Trauma Surgery, University Hospital of Poitiers, 86000 Poitiers, France
4. Department of Pediatric Orthopedics, Cohen Children's Medical Center, Northwell Health, New Hyde Park, New York, NY 11040, USA
* Correspondence: anne.tabard@hcuge.ch
† These authors contributed equally to this work.

Citation: Bazin, L.; Ansorge, A.; Vendeuvre, T.; Cochard, B.; Tabard-Fougère, A.; Vazquez, O.; De Marco, G.; Sarwahi, V.; Dayer, R. Minimally Invasive Surgery for Posterior Spinal Instrumentation and Fusion in Adolescent Idiopathic Scoliosis: Current Status and Future Application. *Children* **2023**, *10*, 1882. https://doi.org/10.3390/children10121882

Academic Editor: Federico Solla

Received: 30 October 2023
Revised: 28 November 2023
Accepted: 29 November 2023
Published: 30 November 2023

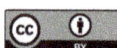

Copyright: © 2023 by the authors. Licensee MDPI, Basel, Switzerland. This article is an open access article distributed under the terms and conditions of the Creative Commons Attribution (CC BY) license (https://creativecommons.org/licenses/by/4.0/).

Abstract: The posterior minimally invasive spine surgery (MISS) approach—or the paraspinal muscle approach—for posterior spinal fusion and segmental instrumentation in adolescent idiopathic scoliosis (AIS) was first reported in 2011. It is less invasive than the traditionally used open posterior midline approach, which is associated with significant morbidity, including denervation of the paraspinal muscles, significant blood loss, and a large midline skin incision. The literature suggests that the MISS approach, though technically challenging and with a longer operative time, provides similar levels of deformity correction, lower intraoperative blood loss, shorter hospital stays, better pain outcomes, and a faster return to sports than the open posterior midline approach. Correction maintenance and fusion rates also seem to be equivalent for both approaches. This narrative review presents the results of relevant publications reporting on spinal segmental instrumentation using pedicle screws and posterior spinal fusion as part of an MISS approach. It then compares them with the results of the traditional open posterior midline approach for treating AIS. It specifically examines perioperative morbidity and radiological and clinical outcomes with a minimal follow-up length of 2 years (range 2–9 years).

Keywords: adolescent idiopathic scoliosis; correction; posterior instrumentation and fusion; paraspinal muscle approach

1. Introduction

Adolescent idiopathic scoliosis (AIS) is the most common spine deformity in the adolescent population. Its prevalence in most populations is about 2.5% [1–4]. Approximately 0.1 to 0.25% of AIS patients eventually undergo surgical treatment when they exceed a certain Cobb angle threshold [1,5,6].

Posterior spinal fusion (PSF) and segmental spinal instrumentation (SSI) using pedicle screws is the most frequently used surgical technique for treating AIS [7,8]. It was first reported by Suk et al. in 1995 and further supported by their later publication (2001) of the first large retrospective series of pediatric deformity cases operated on using this technique and an open posterior midline approach [9,10]. At that time, it was rarely used because of fears of causing neurological damage secondary to poorly positioned pedicle screws. Suk et al.'s series included 462 patients with a deformity (330 idiopathic scoliosis cases) who were operated on using 4604 pedicle screws [9]. As no significant neurological or visceral complications adversely affecting the long-term outcomes were observed, they considered the technique to be reliable and safe. It was associated with significant deformity correction (72%) and reliable correction maintenance (1% correction loss). Posterior segmental pedicle screw instrumentation gained popularity in the 2000s, as evidence was showing the superiority of deformity correction and maintenance of correction, leading to reduced revision surgeries and reduced need to perform additional anterior release surgeries for correcting large curves when compared to previous fixation techniques, like hook-based instrumentations [5,8,11,12].

Ten years later, Sarwahi et al. published a surgical technique paper including two case reports of AIS patients operated on using a posterior paraspinal muscle approach through three small skin incisions—the minimally invasive spine surgery (MISS) approach—to perform PSF and SSI using pedicle screws [13]. As the two initial cases of AIS reported by Sarwahi et al. seemed to reach coronal and sagittal deformity corrections comparable to PSF and standard open SSI, MISS appeared to be a feasible surgical option. They hypothesized multiple potential advantages associated with using this new posterior MISS approach compared to the routine open posterior midline approach, including less blood loss, shorter hospital length of stay, less pain, and the concurrent need for less pain medication, based on the emerging evidence supporting minimal invasive spine surgery for treating adult spine deformities [14,15].

Since MISS for AIS was first introduced in 2011, multiple case series and comparative series, as well as two meta-analyses, evaluated the degree of deformity correction and the potential advantages of this technique in comparison to the traditional open posterior midline approach [13,16–30].

However, not all the relevant available evidence has been comprehensively summarized in a review until now. Therefore, this narrative review describes the posterior MISS approach for performing PSF and SSI on AIS patients and compares its perioperative morbidity and radiological and clinical outcomes with those obtained using the traditional open posterior midline approach. The majority of the cited studies do not select specific Lenke types of curves. Should this be the case, it is explicitly stated where appropriate.

2. Surgical Technique

Wiltse et al. first described the paraspinal muscle approach in 1968 [31]. In 1988, they reported changes to their approach in order to use it for treating additional conditions such as lumbar disc herniations, spinal stenosis and spondylolisthesis in adult patients [32]. The original Wiltse approach involved two paramedian skin incisions with bilateral paramedian incisions of the thoracolumbar fascia and bilateral blunt dissections to separate the multifidus and longissimus muscles. This approach allows for direct access to the lumbar spine's articular processes, laminas, pars interarticularis, and transverse processes.

To minimize skin disruption for cosmetic reasons, this soft-tissue-sparing approach was modified by Sarwahi et al. for use in AIS patients [24]. Instead of using two long paramedian skin incisions, three shorter midline skin incisions are made. The locations of these incisions are determined by the deformity and the resulting preoperative plan for pedicle screw positioning. Fluoroscopy is used preoperatively to mark the incision locations on the skin surface (Figure 1a). Usually, two to five vertebrae are instrumented through each skin incision, and one to two vertebrae are left with no instrumentation between them. Subcutaneous fat in the thoracic region is sharply dissected along the midline, the trapezius muscle, and the latissimus dorsi muscle. The rhomboid minor and major muscles, together with their fascial attachments, are separated from the spinous processes and retracted laterally to allow for a paramedian incision in the thoracolumbar fascia. The extent to which these superficial muscles need to be sharply dissected depends on the exact location of the three incisions and the number of levels to be instrumented and fused. Subcutaneous fat in the lumbar region is directly undermined laterally to allow for a paramedian incision in the thoracolumbar fascia. This is followed by a blunt muscle-sparing approach used to reach the lumbar spine's facet joints—the transverse processes in the thoracic spine (Figure 1b). Gelpi retractors are usually used for this approach, but some surgeons use tubular retractors; both techniques permit delicate muscle dissection and are believed to be equivalent [33]. Ultimately, the posterior elements are exposed from the base of the laminas to the transverse processes using electrocautery. The exposure described here can only be performed on one side at a time. It is followed by the performance of ipsilateral wide facetectomies, with cartilage removal using a bone chisel or a high-speed burr, cannulation of the ipsilateral pedicles using the freehand technique, and the insertion of pedicle markers into the pedicle channels. These steps are then repeated on the other side. If computerized tomography (CT)-based navigation is used instead of the routinely used freehand technique, the posterior bony elements do not need to be exposed using electrocautery [25]. A mixture of autografts from the facetectomies and freeze-dried allograft bone is then applied over the decorticated facet joints. The facet joints between the skin incisions are also decorticated and fused on both sides. Next, the pedicle markers are replaced by pedicle screws using guide wires on one side (the convex side of the major curve is usually addressed first), and then a cobalt–chrome rod, contoured to reproduce the appropriate thoracic kyphosis and lumbar lordosis, is inserted into the reduction tubes fixed on the pedicle screw heads (Figure 2). Depending on the surgeon's preference, the rod can be inserted caudally to reduce the risk of intrusion into the spinal canal or cephalad to avoid inadvertently pushing on the patient's head. Gradual spine-to-rod reduction, using reduction tubes, is used to correct most of the deformity. When additional deformity correction is needed, an additional direct apical segmental derotation is then performed. After the rod's definitive fixation to the screw heads, the reduction tubes are removed. The opposite side is than similarly instrumented. If the amount of correction still needs to be increased at this point, adequately contouring the second rod might enable additional deformity correction through spine-to-rod reduction. Finally, the paraspinal muscle approach is sutured using a routine layered technique. In 2019, Urbanski et al. reported a modification of the paraspinal muscle approach which further reduced soft tissue disruption [25]. Their technique used percutaneous, trans-muscular stab incisions to access the pedicle entry points. As no posterior bony landmarks are exposed, this technique requires CT-based navigation. The latter technique is known to achieve higher pedicle screw placement accuracy and exposes the patients to roughly four times more radiation than the freehand technique (effective dose between 1.11 and 1.48 mSv versus 0.17 and 0.34 mSV), while the rates of pedicle screw misplacement-related complications (0–1.4%) are similar for both techniques [34–39].

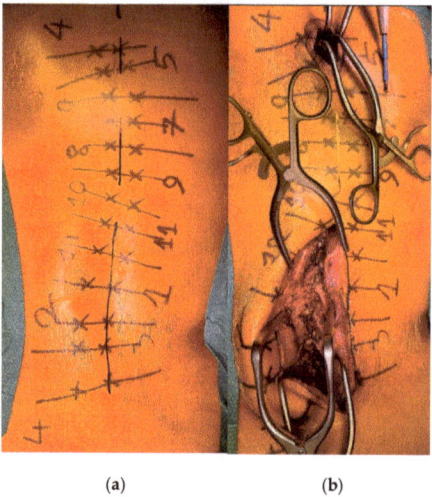

(a) (b)

Figure 1. (a) Preoperative skin marking of the vertebrae, the pedicles, and the three skin incisions. (b) MISS exposure performed on the left lumbar area, with exposure of the facet joints.

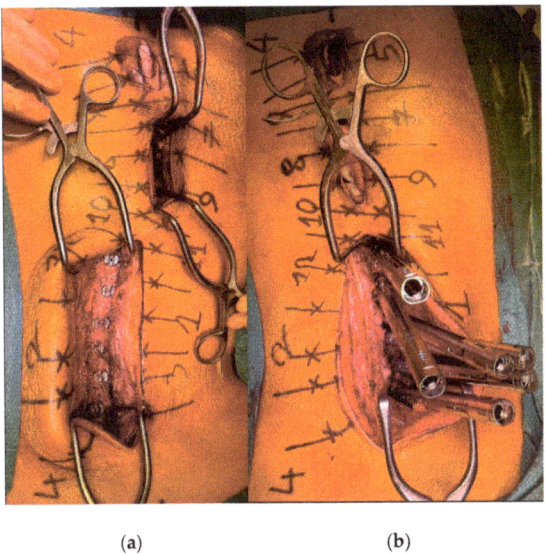

(a)   (b)

Figure 2. (a) The pedicle screws are in place. (b) The reduction tubes are fixed on the pedicle screw heads.

Another modification of the paraspinal muscle approach was reported by Sarwahi et al. in 2023. Its only change involved replacing the three skin incisions with a single, longer skin incision. Compared to the three-incision paraspinal muscle approach (the original MISS), the operative time was shorter and the advantages over an open posterior midline approach were maintained [30].

3. Deformity Correction and Fusion

3.1. Coronal Correction

Most reports support the view that performing SSI and PSF with pedicle screws using a posterior MISS approach results in coronal deformity corrections that do not differ significantly from those obtained using a standard posterior midline approach (see Table 1) [23–28,30]. The best available evidence for this view is the 2022 meta-analysis by Yang et al. [30] They analyzed five comparative series for this parameter, including 713 patients, and found a weighted mean difference (WMD) of −0.01 (95% CI −0.03 to 0.01; $p = 0.518$) [30]. The follow-up (FU) lengths of these series varied between 2 and 9 years.

However, three moderately-sized comparative retrospective series have been inconsistent with this view. The first was published by Miyanji et al. in 2015 and included 46 AIS cases with an FU length of 2 years [23]. It reported a coronal curve correction rate of 58% in the MISS group and 68% in the open posterior midline approach group ($p < 0.001$). The authors thought that this correction difference might be explained by the new technique's learning curve effect. The second series, including 49 patients, was published by Yang et al. in 2021. It found a statistically significant approach-related difference in the coronal major curve correction of 5% ($p = 0.017$) and an approach-related postoperative major curve Cobb angle difference of 3° [26]. A correction curve difference of 3° might not be clinically significant or related to the selected approach, but rather to the correction technique used. Indeed, monoaxial screws with direct apical vertebral derotation were used in conjunction with the open posterior midline approach, but polyaxial screws with spine-to-rod translation were the only reduction technique used in conjunction with the MISS approach. The third series, including 82 patients with Lenke type 1 curves, was described by Syundyukov et al. in 2023 [40]. The coronal major curve correction was significantly greater in the open posterior midline group than in the MISS group when expressed in percentage terms (88% vs. 78%; $p < 0.001$), but not when expressed in degrees (40.5° vs. 46.7°; $p = 0.005$).

Table 1. Coronal major curve correction rates (%) among AIS patients who underwent posterior SSI and PSF using MISS or the open posterior midline approach.

Authors	Year	Study Design	No. of Cases	MISS (%)	OM (%)	p-Value
Miyanji et al. [22]	2013	Pros. comp.	32	63	68	n/a [a]
Miyanji et al. [23]	2015	Retro. comp.	46	58	68	0.001
Sarwahi et al. [24]	2016	Retro. comp.	22	79	85	0.503
Urbanski et al. [25]	2019	Retro. comp.	8	68 [b]	78	0.072
Yang et al. [26]	2021	Retro. comp.	49	65	70	0.017
Si et al. [27]	2021	Retro. comp.	112	65	64	0.862
Sarwahi et al. [28]	2021	Retro. comp.	485	69	68	0.46
Syundyukov et al. [40]	2023	Retro. comp.	82	78	88	<0.001
Sarwahi et al. [41]	2023	Retro. comp.	532	69 or 62 [c]	68	0.49
Yang et al. [30]	2022	Meta-analysis	713	n/a [d]		0.518

The references number [25,27,40], specifically selected Lenke curves type 5C, 1-4, respectively 1. AIS = adolescent idiopathic scoliosis; SSI = segmental spinal instrumentation; PSF = posterior spinal fusion; MISS = minimally invasive spinal surgery; No. = number; OM = open posterior midline approach; pros. comp. = prospective comparative series; retro. comp. = retrospective comparative series; n/a = not available; CI = confidence interval; [a] = not statistically significant (95% CI −0.12 to 0.04); [b] = modified MISS technique using a single midline skin incision instead of three and fascial stab incisions for performing CT-navigated SSI; [c] = 69% correction rate using the original MISS technique with three midline skin incisions or 62% correction rate using the modified MISS technique with a single midline skin incision. [d] = correction rates expressed as a WMD of −0.01; 95% CI −0.03 to 0.001.

3.2. Sagittal Correction

When treating AIS cases, spine surgeons have traditionally focused mainly on correcting coronal deformities [42]. Over the last 20 years, evidence has grown concerning the importance of the physiological sagittal balance, which is necessary to maintain a pain-free erect posture. Consequently, more attention is now given to restoring the patient's physiological sagittal profile, and particularly to correcting the typically encountered thoracic hypokyphosis present with major thoracic curves [42–45]. The two first comparative series, published by Miyanji et al. and Sarwahi et al., reported no significant differences in sagittal deformity correction between their MISS and open posterior midline approach groups [23,24]. Interestingly, the five studies included in Yang et al.'s meta-analysis, which evaluated the sagittal correction, revealed a significant difference in the correction rate for thoracic kyphosis [30]. At their last follow-up, which varied between 2 and 9 years, the pooled MISS and the pooled open posterior midline groups had mean thoracic kyphosis values of 25.80° and 22.71°, respectively. This difference appeared to be especially significant among patients with more than 10 levels fused. In a comparative study including 485 AIS cases with a minimal FU length of 2 years (range of 2–5 years), Sarwahi et al. again found a significantly greater kyphosis correction among MISS patients than among open posterior midline approach patients (kyphosis increase of 17.9% versus −5.3%; $p = 0.007$) [28]. This finding is difficult to explain. It might be related to better preservation of the paraspinal muscles and the posterior ligament complex, which resist the lordosing effect of the direct apical vertebral derotation technique that is often used to correct scoliosis. Indeed, the major forces applied during this maneuver push the thoracic hump ventrally to decrease the rotational deformity and concomitantly induce a reduction in the thoracic kyphosis, as previously reported by Sudo et al. [45]. This explanation, however, contradicts the general understanding that an extensive posterior release enables better restoration of kyphosis [28].

Only the 2023 case series described by Syundykov et al. found a significantly better correction of thoracic hypokyphosis using the open posterior midline approach than using the MISS approach [40]. Their series of 82 patients with Lenke type 1 curves showed a mean increase in the thoracic kyphosis of 4° using the open posterior midline approach and a mean decrease of 4° using the MISS approach. They related the better thoracic kyphosis correction obtained using the midline approach to its better access to the facet joints and to the more extensive ligamentous release.

In summary, there is more evidence supporting the MISS approach as the best one for thoracic kyphosis restoration.

3.3. Fusion Rate

In clinical practice, fusion assessment is usually performed following an analysis of anteroposterior and lateral standing whole-spine radiographs, as routinely performing CT scans would expose adolescents to unnecessarily high doses of radiation. In cases of significant postoperative back pain, with or without radiological signs of pseudarthrosis, a CT scan is usually performed for a more detailed assessment of fusion status and possible implant-related complications. In 1994, Bridwell et al. described a fusion status classification based on standing X-rays (anteroposterior and lateral views) that is still commonly used in research articles [46]. They rated the fusion mass as "definitely solid" (with heavy trabeculations seen along the whole length of the fusion), "probably solid" (meaning there was no evidence of instrumentation failure or a loss of correction, but that mature trabeculation could not be identified at every level), or as "definite pseudarthrosis" (defined as instrumentation failure or a loss of correction greater than 10°, or visible pseudarthrosis).

In a recent comparative study by Yang et al. [33], fusion rates were assessed after a mean FU length of 22 months (range 18–38 months) using Bridwell's classification rating on 86 AIS patients operated on using either an open posterior midline approach with SSI and posterior fusion with allografts or an MISS approach. The MISS group was divided into three subgroups based on the bone substitute used: allograft versus demineralized bone matrix versus demineralized cancellous bone chips. CT scans were only performed on patients with back pain or neurological abnormalities, and were also reviewed to determine fusion status. A "definitely solid" or "probably solid" fusion was achieved in 83% of the MISS group patients and 97% of the posterior midline approach group patients ($p = 0.07$). The bone substitute type which was used did not significantly influence the fusion rate in the three MISS subgroups (85% for allograft, 100% for demineralized bone matrix, and 100% for demineralized cancellous bone chips; $p = 0.221$).

In their meta-analysis, Yang et al. noted the diversity of patients in terms of their curve types and fusion levels across the various studies [30]. Some studies focused on specific Lenke types, while others included a mix of curve types (Lenke types 1–6), and the fusion levels ranged widely from 5 to 12. This heterogeneity complicates direct comparisons of fusion success according to the approach used. Despite these complexities, the occurrence of hardware failures, such as screw or rod breakage, was not significantly different between the MISS and open posterior midline approach groups. This suggests that both approaches can achieve comparably high levels of hardware stability and fusion rates.

4. Perioperative Morbidity

4.1. Estimated Blood Loss and Allogeneic Transfusion Rate

Correcting AIS using SSI and PSF by means of an open posterior midline approach is associated with extensive subperiosteal preparation and a large wound surface. In contrast, the posterior paraspinal muscle approach—the MISS approach—is associated with much less soft tissue disruption. It might, therefore, significantly decrease the mean estimated blood loss (EBL) and the need for allogeneic blood transfusions. Multiple comparative studies have indeed shown significantly lower EBL when using MISS than when using an open posterior midline approach (see Table 2). For instance, in their series of eight AIS cases with Lenke type 5C curves, Urbanski et al. reported a mean EBL of 138 mL when using MISS versus 450 mL (p = 0.016) when using the open posterior midline approach [25]. Their particular low EBL might have been associated with their use of CT-navigation in conjunction with fascial stab incisions, allowing for further minimization of soft tissue disruption, as no bony landmarks needed to be exposed. Yang et al.'s comparative series, including 49 AIS patients, reported a much higher mean EBL with both techniques, but their MISS group still had a significantly lower mean EBL than their open posterior midline group (1279 mL versus 2503 mL, respectively; p < 0.001) [26]. In 2023, Sarwahi et al. reported a large comparative series of 532 AIS cases operated on using either an open posterior midline approach (294 cases), the original three-incision MISS approach (179 cases), or a modified MISS approach known as single long-incision minimally (SLIM) invasive surgery (59 cases) [41]. The mean EBL for the open posterior midline approach group (500 mL) was significantly higher than for the two other groups (302 mL versus 325 mL, respectively; p < 0.00001). The allogeneic transfusion rate (19% versus 5.6% versus 6.8%, respectively; p = 0.001) was also significantly higher for the open posterior midline approach group than for the two other groups. Interestingly, the original MISS group and the SLIM group had comparable mean EBL values (302 mL versus 325 mL, respectively) and allogeneic transfusion rates (5.6% versus 6.8%), suggesting that the extent of the approach-related muscle dissection is more closely associated with the amount of blood loss than the skin incision length. The strongest current evidence corroborating the lower mean EBL when using MISS can be found in Yang et al.'s 2022 meta-analysis, which included six studies and a total of 767 patients [30]. They reported a mean EBL of 288 mL for the MISS group versus 517 mL for the open posterior midline approach group. The same meta-analysis also reported a significantly lower allogeneic blood transfusion rate in the MISS group than in the open posterior midline approach group (8.0% versus 35.0%, respectively; p < 0.001) when analyzing the pooled results of the four studies they included to provide data on allogeneic transfusions.

Table 2. Mean EBL (ml) among AIS patients who underwent posterior SSI and PSF using MISS or the open posterior midline approach.

Authors	Year	Study Design	No. of Cases	MISS (mL)	OM (mL)	p-Value
Miyanji et al. [22]	2013	Pros. comp.	32	277	388	n/a [a]
Miyanji et al. [23]	2015	Retro. comp.	46	261.5	471.1	0.000
Sarwahi et al. [24]	2016	Retro. comp.	22	600	800	0.051
Urbanski et al. [25]	2019	Retro. comp.	8	138.75 [b]	450	0.016
Yang et al. [26]	2021	Retro. comp.	49	1279	2503	<0.001
Si et al. [27]	2021	Retro. comp.	112	502	808	<0.001
Sarwahi et al. [28]	2021	Retro. comp.	485	300	500	<0.001
Alhammoud et al. [29]	2022	Meta-analysis	107	271.1	527	0.019
Syundyukov et al. [40]	2023	Retro. comp.	82	208.7	564.3	<0.001
Sarwahi et al. [41]	2023	Retro. comp.	532	302 vs. 325 [c]	500	0.005
Yang et al. [30]	2023	Meta-analysis	767	n/a [d]		<0.001

The references number [25,27,40], specifically selected Lenke curves type 5C, 1-4, respectively 1. EBL = estimated blood loss; ml = milliliter; AIS = adolescent idiopathic scoliosis; SSI = segmental spinal instrumentation; PSF = posterior spinal fusion; MISS = minimally invasive spinal surgery; No. = number; OM = open posterior midline approach; pros. comp. = prospective comparative series; retro. comp. = retrospective comparative series; n/a = not available; CI = confidence interval; [a] = statistically significant difference: (95% CI −2.6 to −0.6); [b] = modified MISS technique using a single midline skin incision instead of three and fascial stab incisions for performing navigated SSI; [c] = 302 mL is related to the original MISS technique with three midline skin incisions; 325 mL is related to the modified MISS technique with a single midline skin incision; [d] = mean EBL expressed as WMD, −218.76; 95% CI −256.41 to 181.11.

4.2. Operative Time

The MISS approach exposes significantly fewer posterior spinal bony landmarks than the open posterior midline approach. This makes MISS more challenging than the open posterior midline approach when using the freehand technique to perform SSI with pedicle screws. Also, because the skin incisions are on the midline and need to be retracted laterally to one side to perform SSI, instrumentation cannot be carried out bilaterally at the same time, as opposed to with the open posterior midline approach. As a consequence, MISS usually requires a significantly longer mean operative time (ORT) (7.4 to 8.98 h) than the open posterior midline approach (5.77 to 7.07 h) [25–28,41]. This was especially true in the first reported series, which was also influenced by the learning curve effect [47]. Indeed, the early series reported by Sarwahi et al. showed much longer ORTs for MISS approaches than for open posterior midline approaches (8.98 versus 7.07 h, respectively; $p = 0.011$), as did Miyanii et al. (475.3 versus 346.4 min, respectively; $p = 0.000$) [13,22]. The meta-analysis by Yang et al. showed consistently longer ORTs (89 min longer) for MISS approaches than for the open posterior midline approach [30]. To address this disadvantage of the original MISS approach, Sarwahi et al. recently developed and reported a modification to it consisting exclusively of the replacement of the three short skin incisions with a single longer skin incision (SLIM). In their comparative series, ORT was reduced to 262 min when using SLIM compared to 302 using the original MISS approach with three short incisions, while the open posterior midline approach's ORT was 258 min [41].

4.3. Postoperative Pain and Average Opioid Consumption

The Scoliosis Research Society 22-item (SRS-22) pain score and the Visual Analogue Scale (VAS) score are the most direct ways to report pain. The degree of postoperative opioid consumption can also be used to report pain indirectly. The first series reporting MISS use for treating AIS did not find a significant decrease in pain when using MISS in comparison to the use of the open posterior midline approach (average VAS score 3.5 versus 3.4, respectively; $p = 0.698$) [24]. In contrast, the majority of later series reported lower VAS scores or better SRS-22 pain scores for MISS than for the open posterior midline approach [26,27,41]. This fact is further supported by the results of the meta-analysis by Yang et al. [30]. Indeed, the pooled results of the five studies reporting it revealed significantly less postoperative pain according to the VAS score (WMD, 0.84; 95% CI 0.03 to 1.64; $p = 0.042$) and the SRS-22 pain score (WMD, 0.53; 95% CI 0.06 to 1.00; $p = 0.02$). The large comparative series reported by Sarwahi et al., including 485 AIS patients, analogously reported lower postoperative opioid consumption in their MISS group than in their open posterior midline approach group ($p < 0.001$) [28].

4.4. Hospital Length of Stay (LOS)

Hospital length of stay (LOS) is an important indirect marker of postoperative pain and function and has significant financial implications. To the best of our knowledge, only the first series of MISS use reported by Sarwahi et al., which included 22 AIS cases, failed to show significantly a shorter LOS for MISS than for the open posterior midline approach ($p = 0.472$), which might be related to the small number of patients or to the learning curve effect [24]. In contrast, later studies have consistently demonstrated otherwise. For example, the comparative series reported by Urbansky et al., which included only Lenke type 5C curves, showed a significantly shorter LOS for MISS (3.75 versus 7 days; $p = 0.043$) [25]. The results of the meta-analysis by Yang et al. further support this finding (WMD, -1.48; 95% CI -2.48 to -0.48; $p = 0.004$) [30]. Sarwahi et al. found no significant difference in LOS between their original MISS technique with three small skin incisions and their more recent modification with one long skin incision (4 days for both techniques; $p = 0.7$). The LOS was still significantly longer for their open posterior midline group (5 days; $p < 0.001$) [41].

4.5. Intraoperative, Perioperative, and Long-Term Complications

Various complications related to the surgical correction of AIS have been defined and reported in the literature. Hariharan et al. reported the largest 10-year prospective follow-up study to evaluate postoperative complications after the surgical treatment of AIS patients [48]. Of the 282 patients included, 195 underwent posterior spinal fusion using an open posterior midline approach. A total of 19 complications occurred in 18 of the 195 patients (9.7% complication rate), with the most prevalent being surgical site infections (37%), followed by adding-on (26%), pulmonary (16%), neurological (11%), instrumentation (5%), and gastrointestinal issues (5%).

When comparing the complication rates after SSI and PSF using either MISS or the open posterior midline approach, the available comparative series found no statistically relevant differences [23,24,26–29,41]. For instance, the largest case–control series, comparing 192 MISS cases to 293 open posterior midline approach cases, showed similar perioperative complication rates ($\leq$30 days) among both groups (3.1% versus 3.8%; $p = 0.81$) [28]. This was also the case with long-term complications (>30 days) (3.6% versus 1.4%; $p = 0.12$) after a minimal FU length of 2 years (range 2–5 years). Likewise, Yang et al. found no significant approach-related complication rate differences in their meta-analysis (RR, 1.13; 95% CI 0.77 to 1.67; $p = 0.521$), which defined surgical site infection, hardware failure, wound dehiscence, pseudarthrosis, and hemothorax as possible complications [30]. Thus, MISS seems to be a safe alternative to the open posterior midline approach.

5. Clinical and Functional Outcomes

The available literature has usually measured clinical and functional outcomes using the SRS-22 questionnaire. At the two-year follow-up point, Miyanji et al. observed no differences in SRS-22 outcome scores between AIS patients operated on using either the open posterior midline or MISS approaches ($p = 0.715$) [23]. Yang et al. found similar findings in their comparative series at a mean FU length of 9.7 versus 4.6 years for their MISS and open posterior midline approach groups, respectively [26]. Their meta-analysis found non-statistically-significant but slightly higher SRS-22 scores for self-image/appearance and overall satisfaction among patients who underwent MISS [30]. In their comparative series, including 112 AIS cases (Lenke type 1–4 curves) with a minimum follow-up of two years, Si et al. observed lower SRS-22 pain scores in the MIS group than in the PSF group ($p = 0.043$), and found no significant differences in the other SRS-22 score components at the last follow-up (31 versus 32 months FU for the MISS and the open posterior midline group, respectively) [27]. Sarwahi et al. matched 50 AIS patients operated on using the original MISS approach, with 50 patients operated on using the modified single-incision MISS approach and 50 patients operated on using the open posterior midline approach [41]. They were matched according to age, sex, body mass index, and number of levels fused. At 5–6 months of follow-up, the three groups' overall SRS-22 questionnaire scores showed no statistical differences. In contrast, the SRS-22 function and activity scores and pain scores were significantly better for the two MISS groups than for the open posterior midline approach group. On the Sports Activity Questionnaire, MISS patients (both groups) were more likely to return to non-contact ($p = 0.0096$) and contact sports ($p = 0.0095$) within 6 months than the patients operated on using the open posterior midline approach. Considering the relevant available reports, MISS seems—at the very least—not to be inferior to the traditional open posterior midline approach in terms of clinical and functional outcomes at 6 months or 2 years of follow-up. The more recent reports, which have analyzed larger patient cohorts, tend to show the MISS approach's superiority over the posterior open midline approach.

6. Conclusions

Segmental spinal instrumentation (SSI) with pedicle screws and posterior spinal fusion (PSF) using an open posterior midline approach is the most commonly used surgical technique to treat adolescent idiopathic scoliosis (AIS). Based on several comparative series including up to 532 patients and a meta-analysis including 767 patients, the newer minimally invasive spinal surgery (MISS) approach, first introduced by Sarwahi et al. in 2011, appears to be an appropriate alternative to the open posterior midline approach for performing SSI and PSF to treat AIS of any Lenke type. The MISS approach has notably been shown to result in equivalent coronal deformity correction, with some evidence supporting better restoration of thoracic kyphosis. MISS also achieves equivalent complication rates and fusion rates. The relevant advantages of MISS over the open posterior midline approach are lower estimated blood loss, lower perioperative allogeneic transfusion rates, less postoperative pain, and a shorter length of stay at the hospital. The clinical and functional outcomes reported for MISS patients at FU lengths varying between 2 and 9 years are at least as good as those obtained using the open posterior midline approach, while some evidence supports a faster return to non-contact and contact sports among MISS patients.

However, the posterior MISS approach also has limitations. As the exposure is restricted in comparison to the traditional posterior midline approach, it is technically more challenging and associated with longer ORT. We, therefore, recommend that surgeons willing to adopt it exclude cases with major curves over 70° or with less than 50% flexibility during the learning curve period. According to Yang et al., which evaluated this learning curve effect in a recent case series including 76 AIS patients, a trained surgeon for conventional open scoliosis surgery needs to operate 46 times using the MISS technique to achieve proficient surgical skills.

Finally, MISS is a safe, effective alternative to the open posterior midline approach and appears to be superior in terms of perioperative morbidity. We, therefore, encourage surgeons to re-evaluate their routine approaches to SSI and PSF in favor of the MISS approach. In this context, using the single-long-incision, minimally (SLIM) invasive surgery technique provides a valid and more easily generalizable alternative. It significantly shortens the total operative time and reduces the technical complexities associated with the original MISS procedure while preserving the other advantages for AIS patients.

Author Contributions: R.D. had the original idea for the study; L.B., A.A., T.V., A.T.-F., O.V., G.D.M. and B.C. conducted the literature research; L.B. and A.A. drafted the manuscript; A.A., R.D., T.V., B.C., A.T.-F., O.V., G.D.M. and V.S. critically revised the paper's content. All authors have read and agreed to the published version of the manuscript.

Funding: This research received no external funding.

Institutional Review Board Statement: Not applicable.

Informed Consent Statement: Not applicable.

Data Availability Statement: Not applicable.

Conflicts of Interest: The authors declare no conflict of interest.

References

1. Asher, M.A.; Burton, D.C. Adolescent Idiopathic Scoliosis: Natural History and Long Term Treatment Effects. *Scoliosis* **2006**, *1*, 2. [CrossRef]
2. Willner, S.; Udén, A. A Prospective Prevalence Study of Scoliosis in Southern Sweden. *Acta Orthop. Scand.* **1982**, *53*, 233–237. [CrossRef]
3. Rogala, E.J.; Drummond, D.S.; Gurr, J. Scoliosis: Incidence and Natural History. A Prospective Epidemiological Study. *J. Bone Jt. Surg. Am.* **1978**, *60*, 173–176. [CrossRef]
4. Luk, K.D.K.; Lee, C.F.; Cheung, K.M.C.; Cheng, J.C.Y.; Ng, B.K.W.; Lam, T.P.; Mak, K.H.; Yip, P.S.F.; Fong, D.Y.T. Clinical Effectiveness of School Screening for Adolescent Idiopathic Scoliosis: A Large Population-Based Retrospective Cohort Study. *Spine* **2010**, *35*, 1607–1614. [CrossRef]
5. Pesenti, S.; Jouve, J.-L.; Morin, C.; Wolff, S.; Sales De Gauzy, J.; Chalopin, A.; Ibnoulkhatib, A.; Polirsztok, E.; Walter, A.; Schuller, S.; et al. Evolution of Adolescent Idiopathic Scoliosis: Results of a Multicenter Study at 20 Years' Follow-Up. *Orthop. Traumatol. Surg. Res.* **2015**, *101*, 619–622. [CrossRef]
6. Cheng, J.C.; Castelein, R.M.; Chu, W.C.; Danielsson, A.J.; Dobbs, M.B.; Grivas, T.B.; Gurnett, C.A.; Luk, K.D.; Moreau, A.; Newton, P.O.; et al. Adolescent Idiopathic Scoliosis. *Nat. Rev. Dis. Primers* **2015**, *1*, 1–21. [CrossRef]

7. Lonner, B.S.; Ren, Y.; Yaszay, B.; Cahill, P.J.; Shah, S.A.; Betz, R.R.; Samdani, A.F.; Shufflebarger, H.L.; Newton, P.O. Evolution of Surgery for Adolescent Idiopathic Scoliosis Over 20 Years: Have Outcomes Improved? *Spine* **2018**, *43*, 402–410. [CrossRef]
8. Block, A.M.; Tamburini, L.M.; Zeng, F.; Mancini, M.R.; Jackson, C.A.; Antonacci, C.L.; Karsmarski, O.P.; Stelzer, J.W.; Wellington, I.J.; Lee, M.C. Surgical Treatment of Pediatric Scoliosis: Historical Origins and Review of Current Techniques. *Bioengineering* **2022**, *9*, 600. [CrossRef]
9. Suk, S.-I.; Kim, W.-J.; Lee, S.-M.; Kim, J.-H.; Chung, E.-R. Thoracic Pedicle Screw Fixation in Spinal Deformities: Are They Really Safe? *Spine* **2001**, *26*, 2049–2057. [CrossRef]
10. Suk, S.I.; Lee, C.K.; Kim, W.J.; Chung, Y.J.; Park, Y.B. Segmental Pedicle Screw Fixation in the Treatment of Thoracic Idiopathic Scoliosis. *Spine* **1995**, *20*, 1399–1405. [CrossRef]
11. Lonner, B.S.; Auerbach, J.D.; Boachie-Adjei, O.; Shah, S.A.; Hosogane, N.; Newton, P.O. Treatment of Thoracic Scoliosis: Are Monoaxial Thoracic Pedicle Screws the Best Form of Fixation for Correction? *Spine* **2009**, *34*, 845–851. [CrossRef]
12. Lonner, B.S.; Auerbach, J.D.; Estreicher, M.B.; Kean, K.E. Thoracic Pedicle Screw Instrumentation: The Learning Curve and Evolution in Technique in the Treatment of Adolescent Idiopathic Scoliosis. *Spine* **2009**, *34*, 2158–2164. [CrossRef]
13. Sarwahi, V.; Wollowick, A.L.; Sugarman, E.P.; Horn, J.J.; Gambassi, M.; Amaral, T.D. Minimally Invasive Scoliosis Surgery: An Innovative Technique in Patients with Adolescent Idiopathic Scoliosis. *Scoliosis* **2011**, *6*, 16. [CrossRef]
14. Anand, N.; Baron, E.M.; Thaiyananthan, G.; Khalsa, K.; Goldstein, T.B. Minimally invasive Multilevel Percutaneous Correction and Fusion for Adult Lumbar Degenerative Scoliosis: A Technique and Feasibility Study. *J. Spinal Disord. Tech.* **2008**, *21*, 459–467. [CrossRef]
15. Dakwar, E.; Cardona, R.F.; Smith, D.A.; Uribe, J.S. Early Outcomes and Safety of the Minimally Invasive, Lateral Retroperitoneal Transpsoas Approach for Adult Degenerative Scoliosis. *Neurosurg. Focus.* **2010**, *28*, E8. [CrossRef]
16. Brodano, G.B.; Martikos, K.; Vommaro, F.; Greggi, T.; Boriani, S. Less Invasive Surgery in Idiopathic Scoliosis: A Case Report. *Eur. Rev. Med. Pharmacol. Sci.* **2014**, *18*, 24–28.
17. De Bodman, C.; Ansorge, A.; Tabard-Fougère, A.; Amirghasemi, N.; Dayer, R. Clinical and Radiological Outcomes of Minimally-Invasive Surgery for Adolescent Idiopathic Scoliosis at a Minimum Two Years' Follow-Up. *Bone Jt. J.* **2020**, *102-B*, 506–512. [CrossRef]
18. De Bodman, C.; Miyanji, F.; Borner, B.; Zambelli, P.-Y.; Racloz, G.; Dayer, R. Minimally Invasive Surgery for Adolescent Idiopathic Scoliosis: Correction of Deformity and Peri-Operative Morbidity in 70 Consecutive Patients. *Bone Jt. J.* **2017**, *99-B*, 1651–1657. [CrossRef]
19. Yang, J.H.; Chang, D.-G.; Suh, S.W.; Damani, N.; Lee, H.-N.; Lim, J.; Mun, F. Safety and Effectiveness of Minimally Invasive Scoliosis Surgery for Adolescent Idiopathic Scoliosis: A Retrospective Case Series of 84 Patients. *Eur. Spine J.* **2020**, *29*, 761–769. [CrossRef]
20. Park, S.C.; Son, S.W.; Yang, J.H.; Chang, D.-G.; Suh, S.W.; Nam, Y.; Kim, H.J. Novel Surgical Technique for Adolescent Idiopathic Scoliosis: Minimally Invasive Scoliosis Surgery. *JCM* **2022**, *11*, 5847. [CrossRef]
21. Samdani, A.F.; Asghar, J.; Miyanji, F.; Haw, J.; Haddix, K. Minimally Invasive Treatment of Pediatric Spinal Deformity. *Semin. Spine Surg.* **2011**, *23*, 72–75. [CrossRef]
22. Amer Samdani, F.M. Minimally Invasive Surgery for AIS: An Early Prospective Comparison with Standard Open Posterior Surgery. *J. Spine* **2013**, *5*, 1. [CrossRef]
23. Miyanji, F.; Desai, S. Minimally Invasive Surgical Options for Adolescent Idiopathic Scoliosis. *Semin. Spine Surg.* **2015**, *27*, 39–44. [CrossRef]
24. Sarwahi, V.; Horn, J.J.; Kulkarni, P.M.; Wollowick, A.L.; Lo, Y.; Gambassi, M.; Amaral, T.D. Minimally Invasive Surgery in Patients With Adolescent Idiopathic Scoliosis: Is It Better than the Standard Approach? A 2-Year Follow-up Study. *Clin. Spine Surg.* **2016**, *29*, 331–340. [CrossRef]
25. Urbanski, W.; Zaluski, R.; Kokaveshi, A.; Aldobasic, S.; Miekisiak, G.; Morasiewicz, P. Minimal invasive posterior correction of Lenke 5C idiopathic scoliosis: Comparative analysis of minimal invasive vs. open surgery. *Arch. Orthop. Trauma. Surg.* **2019**, *139*, 1203–1208. [CrossRef]
26. Yang, J.H.; Kim, H.J.; Chang, D.-G.; Suh, S.W. Comparative Analysis of Radiologic and Clinical Outcomes Between Conventional Open and Minimally Invasive Scoliosis Surgery for Adolescent Idiopathic Scoliosis. *World Neurosurg.* **2021**, *151*, e234–e240. [CrossRef]
27. Si, G.; Li, T.; Wang, Y.; Liu, X.; Li, C.; Yu, M. Minimally Invasive Surgery versus Standard Posterior Approach for Lenke Type 1–4 Adolescent Idiopathic Scoliosis: A Multicenter, Retrospective Study. *Eur. Spine J.* **2021**, *30*, 706–713. [CrossRef]
28. Sarwahi, V.; Galina, J.M.; Hasan, S.; Atlas, A.; Ansorge, A.; De Bodman, C.; Lo, Y.; Amaral, T.D.; Dayer, R. Minimally Invasive Versus Standard Surgery in Idiopathic Scoliosis Patients: A Comparative Study. *Spine* **2021**, *46*, 1326–1335. [CrossRef]
29. Alhammoud, A.; Alborno, Y.; Baco, A.M.; Othman, Y.A.; Ogura, Y.; Steinhaus, M.; Sheha, E.D.; Qureshi, S.A. Minimally Invasive Scoliosis Surgery Is a Feasible Option for Management of Idiopathic Scoliosis and Has Equivalent Outcomes to Open Surgery: A Meta-Analysis. *Glob. Spine J.* **2022**, *12*, 483–492. [CrossRef]
30. Yang, H.; Jia, X.; Hai, Y. Posterior Minimally Invasive Scoliosis Surgery versus the Standard Posterior Approach for the Management of Adolescent Idiopathic Scoliosis: An Updated Meta-Analysis. *J. Orthop. Surg. Res.* **2022**, *17*, 58. [CrossRef]
31. Wiltse, L.L.; Bateman, J.G.; Hutchinson, R.H.; Nelson, W.E. The Paraspinal Sacrospinalis-Splitting Approach to the Lumbar Spine. *JBJS* **1968**, *50*, 919. [CrossRef]

32. Wiltse, L.L.; Spencer, C.W. New Uses and Refinements of the Paraspinal Approach to the Lumbar Spine. *Spine* **1988**, *13*, 696–706. [CrossRef]
33. Yang, J.H. Fusion Rates Based on Type of Bone Graft Substitute Using Minimally Invasive Scoliosis Surgery for Adolescent Idiopathic Scoliosis. *BMC Musculoskelet. Disord.* **2023**, *24*, 30. [CrossRef]
34. Li, G.; Lv, G.; Passias, P.; Kozanek, M.; Metkar, U.S.; Liu, Z.; Wood, K.B.; Rehak, L.; Deng, Y. Complications Associated with Thoracic Pedicle Screws in Spinal Deformity. *Eur. Spine J.* **2010**, *19*, 1576–1584. [CrossRef]
35. Upendra, B.N.; Meena, D.; Chowdhury, B.; Ahmad, A.; Jayaswal, A. Outcome-Based Classification for Assessment of Thoracic Pedicular Screw Placement. *Spine* **2008**, *33*, 384–390. [CrossRef]
36. Welch, N.; Mota, F.; Birch, C.; Hutchinson, L.; Hedequist, D. Robotics Coupled With Navigation for Pediatric Spine Surgery: Initial Intraoperative Experience With 162 Cases. *J. Pediatr. Orthop.* **2023**, *43*, e337–e342. [CrossRef]
37. Berlin, C.; Quante, M.; Thomsen, B.; Koeszegvary, M.; Platz, U.; Ivanits, D.; Halm, H. Intraoperative Radiation Exposure to Patients in Idiopathic Scoliosis Surgery with Freehand Insertion Technique of Pedicle Screws and Comparison to Navigation Techniques. *Eur. Spine J.* **2020**, *29*, 2036–2045. [CrossRef]
38. Dabaghi Richerand, A.; Christodoulou, E.; Li, Y.; Caird, M.S.; Jong, N.; Farley, F.A. Comparison of Effective Dose of Radiation During Pedicle Screw Placement Using Intraoperative Computed Tomography Navigation Versus Fluoroscopy in Children With Spinal Deformities. *J. Pediatr. Orthop.* **2016**, *36*, 530–533. [CrossRef]
39. Su, A.W.; McIntosh, A.L.; Schueler, B.A.; Milbrandt, T.A.; Winkler, J.A.; Stans, A.A.; Larson, A.N. How Does Patient Radiation Exposure Compare With Low-Dose O-Arm Versus Fluoroscopy for Pedicle Screw Placement in Idiopathic Scoliosis? *J. Pediatr. Orthop.* **2017**, *37*, 171–177. [CrossRef]
40. Syundyukov, A.R.; Nikolaev, N.S.; Vissarionov, S.V.; Kornyakov, P.N.; Bhandarkar, K.S.; Emelianov, V.U. Less Correction with Minimally Invasive Surgery for Adolescent Idiopathic Scoliosis Compared to Open Surgical Correction. *J. Child. Orthop.* **2023**, *17*, 141–147. [CrossRef]
41. Sarwahi, V.; Visahan, K.; Hasan, S.; Patil, A.; Grunfeld, M.; Atlas, A.; Galina, J.; Ansorge, A.; Lo, Y.; Amaral, T.D.; et al. SLIM: Single Long-Incision Minimally Invasive Surgery. *Spine* **2023**, epub ahead of print. [CrossRef]
42. Newton, P.O.; Yaszay, B.; Upasani, V.V.; Pawelek, J.B.; Bastrom, T.P.; Lenke, L.G.; Lowe, T.; Crawford, A.; Betz, R.; Lonner, B.; et al. Preservation of Thoracic Kyphosis Is Critical to Maintain Lumbar Lordosis in the Surgical Treatment of Adolescent Idiopathic Scoliosis. *Spine* **2010**, *35*, 1365–1370. [CrossRef]
43. Bridwell, K.H. Surgical Treatment of Idiopathic Adolescent Scoliosis. *Spine* **1999**, *24*, 2607–2616. [CrossRef]
44. Majdouline, Y.; Aubin, C.-E.; Robitaille, M.; Sarwark, J.F.; Labelle, H. Scoliosis Correction Objectives in Adolescent Idiopathic Scoliosis. *J. Pediatr. Orthop.* **2007**, *27*, 775–781. [CrossRef]
45. Sudo, H.; Abe, Y.; Kokabu, T.; Ito, M.; Abumi, K.; Ito, Y.M.; Iwasaki, N. Correlation Analysis between Change in Thoracic Kyphosis and Multilevel Facetectomy and Screw Density in Main Thoracic Adolescent Idiopathic Scoliosis Surgery. *Spine J.* **2016**, *16*, 1049–1054. [CrossRef]
46. Bridwell, K.H.; O'Brien, M.F.; Lenke, L.G.; Baldus, C.; Blanke, K. Posterior Spinal Fusion Supplemented with Only Allograft Bone in Paralytic Scoliosis. Does It Work? *Spine* **1994**, *19*, 2658–2666. [CrossRef]
47. Yang, J.H.; Kim, H.J.; Chang, D.-G.; Nam, Y.; Suh, S.W. Learning Curve for Minimally Invasive Scoliosis Surgery in Adolescent Idiopathic Scoliosis. *World Neurosurg.* **2023**, *175*, e201–e207. [CrossRef]
48. Hariharan, A.R.; Shah, S.A.; Petfield, J.; Baldwin, M.; Yaszay, B.; Newton, P.O.; Lenke, L.G.; Lonner, B.S.; Miyanji, F.; Sponseller, P.D.; et al. Complications Following Surgical Treatment of Adolescent Idiopathic Scoliosis: A 10-Year Prospective Follow-up Study. *Spine Deform.* **2022**, *10*, 1097–1105. [CrossRef]

Disclaimer/Publisher's Note: The statements, opinions and data contained in all publications are solely those of the individual author(s) and contributor(s) and not of MDPI and/or the editor(s). MDPI and/or the editor(s) disclaim responsibility for any injury to people or property resulting from any ideas, methods, instructions or products referred to in the content.

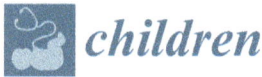

Brief Report

Feasibility, Safety and Reliability of Surgeon-Directed Transcranial Motor Evoked Potentials Monitoring in Scoliosis Surgery

Aude Kerdoncuff [1], Patrice Henry [2], Roxane Compagnon [1], Franck Accadbled [1], Jérôme Sales de Gauzy [1] and Tristan Langlais [1,*]

1 Department of Paediatric Orthopedic Surgery, Children's Hospital, Toulouse University, 31062 Toulouse, France; kerdoncuffa@outlook.fr (A.K.); roxane.compagnon@gmail.com (R.C.); accadbled.f@chu-toulouse.fr (F.A.); salesdegauzy.j@chu-toulouse.fr (J.S.d.G.)
2 Department of Neurology, Purpan Hospital, Toulouse University, 31062 Toulouse, France; henry.p@chu-toulouse.fr
* Correspondence: langlais.t@chu-toulouse.fr

Abstract: (1) Background: Neuromonitoring is essential in corrective surgery for scoliosis. Our aim was to assess the feasibility, safety and reliability of "surgeon-directed" intraoperative monitoring transcranial motor evoked potentials (MEP) of patients. (2) Methods: A retrospective single-center study of a cohort of 190 scoliosis surgeries, monitored by NIM ECLIPSE (Medtronic), between 2017 and 2021. Girls (144) and boys (46) (mean age of 15 years) were included. There were 149 idiopathic and 41 secondary scoliosis. The monitoring consisted of stimulating the primary motor cortex to record the MEP with muscular recording on the thenar, vastus lateralis, tibialis anterior and adductor hallucis muscles. (3) Results: The monitoring data was usable in 180 cases (94.7%), with 178 true negatives, no false negatives and one false positive. There was one true positive case. The predictive negative value was 100%. The monitoring data was unusable in 10 cases (i.e., three idiopathic and seven secondary scoliosis). (4) Conclusions: Simplified transcranial MEP monitoring known as "surgeon-directed module" is usable, safety and reliable in surgery for moderate scoliosis. It is feasible in 95% of cases with a negative predictive value of 100%.

Keywords: scoliosis; multimodal spinal cord intra operative monitoring; pediatric spinal surgery; complex spine deformities

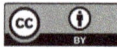

1. Introduction

Scoliosis surgery carries a risk of neurological complications estimated at between 0.35% and 1% of cases [1–3]. This complication rate can be as high as 9% in certain congenital deformities [4]. Intraoperative neuromonitoring is necessary to reduce this risk [5] and has been recommended by the SRS since 1992 [6]. Several monitoring methods have been proposed, but the gold standard is multimodal monitoring, which analyzes somesthetic evoked potentials (SEPs) and motor evoked potentials (MEPs) performed by a doctor specializing in electrophysiology [7]. SEPs were described in the 1970s and assess the ascending sensory pathways whereas MEPs were described in the 1980s and directly analyze the descending motor pathways [8]. MEP procedure uses electrical or magnetic stimulation of the cortex or spinal cord to produce signals in the corticospinal pathways [8]. Some teams [9,10] combine the two techniques (MEPs and SEPs) to achieve reliable neuromonitoring. However, most teams do not have a permanent electrophysiologist due to a lack of resources and funding. To compensate for the lack of electrophysiologists, simplified monitoring techniques (i.e., MEPs only)—known as surgeon-directed modules—have recently been developed that are easy to use and interpret [11,12]. They allow the surgical team to perform neurological monitoring in the absence of an electrophysiologist. The aim of our study was to assess the feasibility, safety and reliability of this surgeon-directed module technique, based on a cohort of scoliosis operations in children, adolescents and young adults.

2. Materials and Methods

2.1. Design and Population Criteria

This is a single-center retrospective study based on the records of operated spinal deformities from 2017 to 2021. The inclusion criteria were idiopathic or secondary scoliosis who underwent a posterior correction-fusion or posterior growing rods and a neuromonitoring performed by the surgeon only. The exclusion criteria were scoliosis surgery with monitoring by an electrophysiologist, corrections of isolated kyphosis or spondylolisthesis, and vertebral fracture treatment. The patient's records monitoring was made possible by the computerized patient file, completed progressively by the referring surgeon. Of the 626 spinal surgical procedures conducted over the inclusion period, the monitoring was surgeon-directed in 190 consecutive cases (Figure 1).

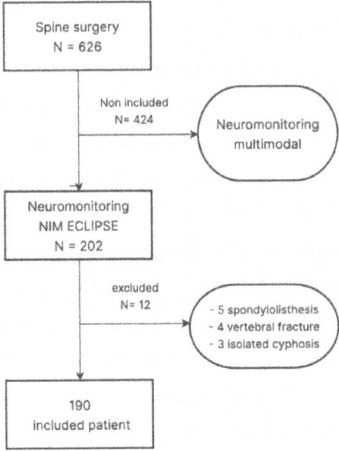

Figure 1. Flow chart.

The mean age was 15 years and 3 months (SD = 3 years, range from 5 to 26 years). The cohort comprised 144 girls and 46 boys. One hundred and forty-nine idiopathic scoliosis and 41 secondary scoliosis were included. This secondary scoliosis included: 14 cerebral palsy, two spinal muscular atrophies, six myopathies, nine congenital deformities (two of which were operated on as part of a poly-malformities syndrome with associated cardiopathy), one Marfan syndrome, one hypophosphatemia rickets, two Prader-Willi syndromes, two arthrogryposis, one Scheuermann disease, two syndromic obesities with hypopituitarism and one neurofibromatosis. The radiographic characteristic of the deformity is reported in Table 1. For the patients included in our cohort, the number of times monitoring had been possible was observed and the number of true and false negatives and true and false positives reported. The tracings were analyzed by the surgeon during the operation and by an electrophysiologist at a distance. Surgeons were trained by the neurophysiologist in the correct positioning of the electrodes, how to monitor them and how to be vigilant for anomalies during the procedure. Monitoring failures at the start of the system's implementation are linked to the learning curve for monitoring. In addition, all patients were operated on by two surgeons specializing in the management of spinal deformities in children (JSDG and FA) and with considerable technique expertise. The surgical technique for spinal arthrodesis depended on the type of curvature. A hybrid construct using at proximal a supra-transverse hook and pedicle hook clamp (or pedicle screw) [13], sublaminar band in the thoracic area [14], and distal lumbar screws in cases of thoracic curvature. In cases of lumbar or thoracotomy-lumbar curvature, an "all-screw" construct was used.

Table 1. Primary radiographic profile of cohort by diagnosis.

Etiology		ADC * Coronal Pre-Operative	Cincinnati Correction Index	ADC * Coronal Post Op
Idiopathic	Average	49	2.17	16
	SD **	15	1.69	10
	Min-max	12–95	0.4–11	0–72
Secondary	Average	60	3.3	29
	SD **	22	3.3	21
	Min-max	23–115	1–18	6–80

* ADC: Cobb angle, ** SD: Standard deviation.

2.2. Neuromonitoring Procedure

Neuromonitoring was conducted using the integrated "surgeon-directed" module on the NIM ECLIPSE device (Medtronic, Minneapolis, MN, USA). Only the integrity of the pyramidal motor pathway is explored by the transcortical electrical stimulation of the primary motor cortex with recording of the motor responses at the distal muscular effectors in the hands and lower limbs. The control panel on the NIM ECLIPSE device displays any faulty connection or other fault. The stimulation parameters (train, number of impulses in the train, interval between each electric shock, etc.) and the reception parameters (bandwidths) are preset by the manufacturer. Only the stimulation intensity and the recorded MEP response signal amplitude can be changed by the surgeon user. The stimulation intensity is gradually increased until satisfactory responses are obtained. It ranges from 150 to 450 volts and rarely exceeds 500 volts. Safety features measure the amperage delivered to the scalp. In our center, we use between 250 and 350 volts on average. The maximum amplitude obtained is specific to each patient and determines the choice of the useful stimulation intensity. There is a great variability between individuals in MEP amplitudes from 0.050 to 500 millivolts and for some muscles and patients' maximum amplitudes of 1 to 4 volts. It is important to adapt the stimulations in young children and patients with seizure, especially if this is poorly controlled, with stimulations that stay low by precaution. After anesthetic induction, the electrodes are positioned by the surgeon before the patient is turned prone (Figure 2). The recording electrodes (muscles) are positioned on the lower limbs (adductor hallucis, tibialis anterior, vastus lateralis muscles) and on the upper limbs (thenar eminence). The stimulation electrodes are positioned on the projection regions on the scalp of the primary motor cortex. As for all electrophysiological procedures, a neutral electrode, known as the "earth ground", must be positioned on one of the iliac crests. The electrodes placed on the upper limbs serve as controls to detect false positives. A first stimulation is conducted before incision with patient under analgesia to obtain a baseline and verify that the monitoring system is functioning correctly (Figure 3). Stimulations are then conducted after each operative phase: at the end of the incision, after positioning the implants, after positioning each rod and at the end of the corrective surgery. In cases of loss of signal (Figure 4), the patient's vital signs and the anesthetic products dispensed are verified with the anesthetist and modified if necessary. If the anomalies persist, a Stagnara Wake up test is performed to assess the patient's active clinical motricity [15].

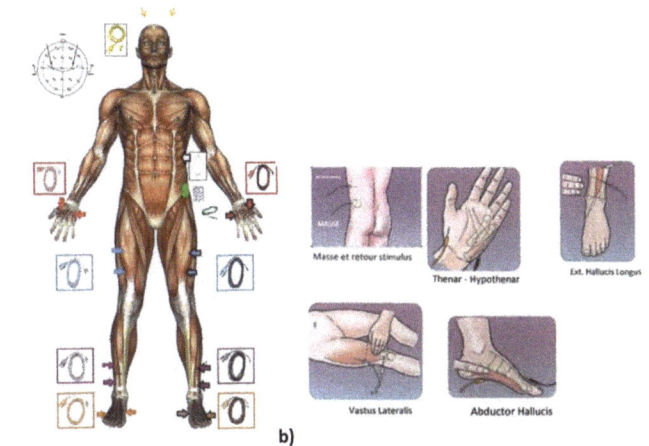

Figure 2. Electrode schemes. (**a**) Electrode sites and color code. Color and white go to right, color and black go to left. Red are thenar sites; blue are vastus lateralis; purple is tibialis anterior; and orange are abductor hallucis. Yellow electrodes go to right and left motor cortex area. The green electrode, called "earth ground", is placed on the iliac crest. (**b**) Focus on each electrode site.

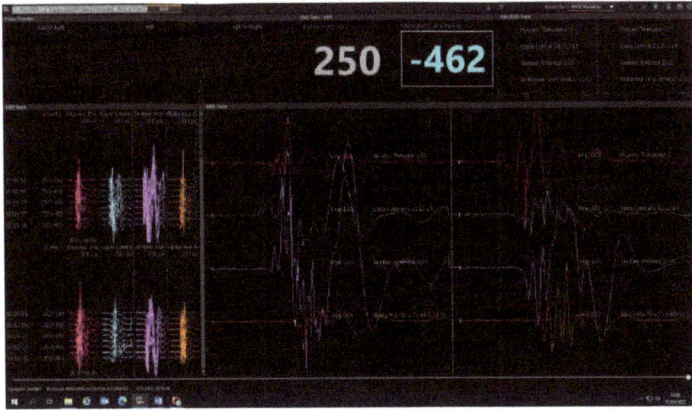

Figure 3. Normal neuromonitoring. Red curves corresponded to the thenar muscular responses; blue curves to the vastus lateralis muscular responses; purple curves to the tibialis anterior muscular responses; and the orange curves to the abductor hallucis muscular responses.

2.3. Statistical Analysis

Demographic and radiographic measure was presented, such as mean, standard deviation (SD) and the range. The number of cases (and percentage) in which monitoring by the surgeon module could be achieved were reported and then analyzed according to the sites where the motor signal was collected. The sensitivity for detecting a potential neurological anomaly by the surgeon direct module MEP is expressed as the percentage value of the ratio of true positives (i.e., one case) to the total number of subjects who had clinically diagnosed neurological abnormalities due to the surgical procedures (i.e., one true positive and none false negative). The specificity is expressed as the percentage value of the ratio of true negatives (i.e., 178 cases) to the total number of subjects who had no clinically diagnosed neurological abnormalities due to the surgical procedures (i.e., 178 true negative + one false positive). The negative predictive value is expressed as the percentage of the ratio of true negatives (178 cases) to the total number of subjects whose neuromonitoring surgeon module did not detect any neurological abnormality (178 true negatives + none false negatives).

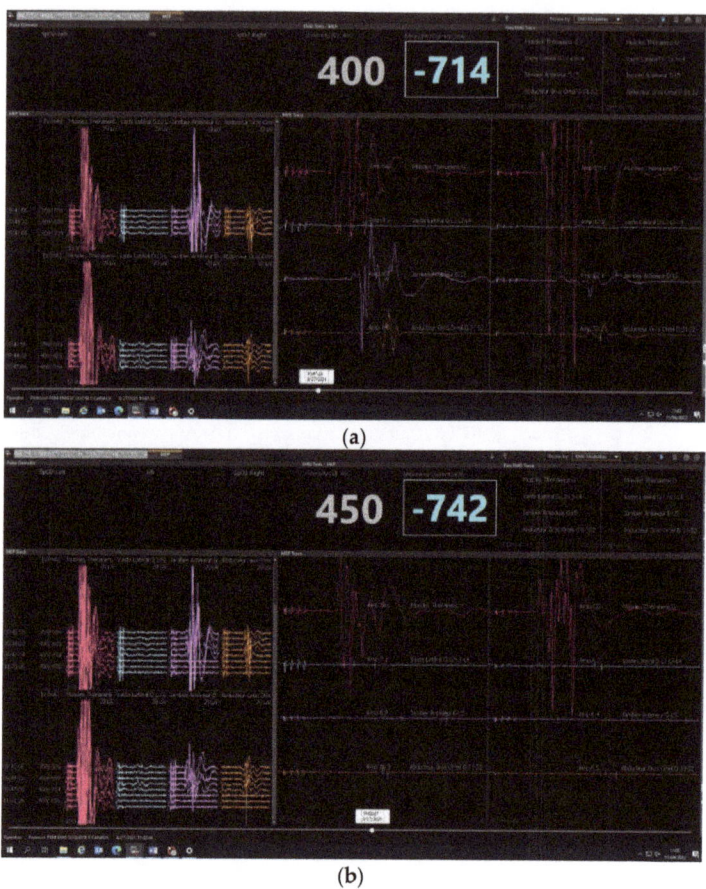

Figure 4. (a) Baseline before incision (b) True positive: Neuromonitoring alert, loss of all responses except upper limb.

3. Results

3.1. Feasibility

The monitoring data was usable in 180 cases (94.7%). It was unusable in 10 cases, either because the response voltages were too low, there was no effective stimulation, there were aberrant responses or there was an initial response only in the upper limbs. This occurred in two idiopathic scoliosis cases that had uninterpretable responses because of an inappropriate anesthesia protocol. These two cases occurred at the beginning of our experience. The other case was an early idiopathic scoliosis with uninterpretable responses due to the immaturity of the nervous system and insufficient cortical stimulation. The other seven cases were secondary scoliosis (five cerebral palsy and two myopathies). Concerning the 180 usable cases, 99 patients (55%) had analyzable and reproducible responses at 8 receptor sites. 60 cases (33%) had responses at 6 of the 8 sites, 13 cases (7%) had responses at 4 of the 8 sites, and 8 cases (5%) had only 2 reproducible and symmetric sites on the lower limbs but with no analyzable response on the upper limbs. The analysis of the responses in function to the muscle group showed that usable responses were more frequent for the tibialis anterior muscle (93% of cases). The vastus lateralis muscle only provided usable responses in 56% of cases. In 85% of cases, we obtained usable responses in the control muscle group (thenar) and in the adductor hallucis group.

3.2. Safety and Reliability Study

The sensitivity for detecting a potential neurological anomaly was 100%, and the specificity was 99%. The predictive negative value was 100%. In the 180 cases where the monitoring data was usable, we found 178 true negatives, no false negatives and one false positive that required a wake-up test with recovery of evoked potentials occurring before the patient was actually awake. There was one true positive case with regressive partial tetraplegia in a patient who had undergone multiple operations. Three patients had a postoperative neurological examination that was not equivalent to their preoperative examination but not detectable by the monitoring (one loss of strength in the upper limbs in myopathy, one L4 radicular sensory deficit, one sensory deficit by compression on early mobilization of the interbody cage). These were not a result of a failure in the monitoring since such anomalies cannot be detected by the monitoring method used.

4. Discussion

To our knowledge, there are two recent publications reporting the results of "surgeon-directed module" NIM ECLIPSE for spinal surgery in children [11,12]. Magampa et al. [11] reviewed 299 cases operated for spinal deformity and using the MEP transcranial surgeon-module as a neurological monitoring tool. 93.3% (versus 94.7% in our paper) had acceptable tracings throughout the operation and woke up with normal clinical neurological function. Also in their study, the negative predictive value was 100%. Their secondary analysis showed that deterioration of motor potentials was significantly higher in congenital scoliosis than in AIS. Chan et al. [12] assessed transcranial MEP surgeon-module in 142 deformity correction surgeries. They also reported a negative predictive value of 100% with three cases (2.11%) showing complete visual loss of signals which led to reversal of the surgical procedure.

Our study supports the results of the two previous studies [11,12]. Surgeon-directed transcranial MEP was feasible in 94.7% of cases (180 out of 190) and provides new information regarding the response of muscle groups to motor stimulation of the cortex. This study shows that in 95% of cases at least four muscle sites have a reliable response among the eight sites tested. Focus on idiopathic scoliosis, surgeon monitoring was feasible in 146 out of 149 cases (i.e., 98% of cases). Of these three cases that could not be performed, two occurred at the start of our experiment with an unsuitable anesthetic protocol. Over the last few years, several risk factors involving modifications to the nerve afferents have been evidenced [16]. Many types of medication can influence the functioning of the motor pathways, notably curare, halogen gas and lidocaine, etc. Conversely, spinal anesthesia (morphine or sufentanil) has no influence on medullary function. The patient's vital signs, notably low blood pressure, can change the electrophysiological responses. These merit attentive surveillance and highlight the crucial need for collaboration with the anesthesia team and the use of a predefined anesthesia protocol.

Concerning secondary scoliosis, surgeon monitoring was feasible in 34 out of 41 cases (i.e., 83% of cases). This difference in etiology was not reported in the two previous articles [11,12]. Recently, Shrader et al. [17] showed that 20.8% of children (among a cohort of 304 cases) with cerebral palsy could not be monitored by transcranial MEPs during spinal arthrodesis surgery. Latency times are often increased in these patients, and the surgeon must be vigilant about the value of the simulation voltage at the risk of triggering an increase in seizure activity [17].

Our study reported one case of false positives and one case of true positives. The steps to follow in cases of MEP disappearance are well defined. First, the patient's vital signs should be checked, as should the drugs being dispensed, which can be modified if necessary. In cases of persistent anomalies, a wake-up test should be conducted. Generally, in the absence of neurological lesions, simply reducing the drugs and maintaining mean arterial pressure (MAP) > 70–80 mm Hg makes it possible to recover satisfactory curves without waiting for the patient to wake up completely. This is called the "anesthetic fade" by Ushirozako et al. [18]. We consider this to be an electrophysiological wake-up test with no actual clinical wake-up.

Previous studies assessed the efficacy of the different neuromonitoring methods (somatosensory evoked potential, motor evoked potential, neurogenic motor evoked potential, D waves and pedicular screw testing) and recommended the multimodal neuromonitoring because it was demonstrated that SSEP had 92% sensitivity and 98% specificity in detecting postoperative neurological complications [9,10,19–21]. This technique makes it possible to use the association of several simultaneous monitoring modalities (for example SSEP and MEP or SSEP and NMEP), in the presence of a neurophysiologist or electrophysiologist. SSEP change from baseline was defined as a 10% increase in latency and/or 50% decrease in amplitude. The MEP change was defined as a modification of the baseline, unilaterally or bilaterally. As our study confirms, using a "surgeon-directed" module is not the most exhaustive surveillance method but the technique makes it possible to eliminate the systematic clinical wake-up test, which provides non-negligible benefits.

Our study has limitations. It is a retrospective study, but no prospective study has been performed in the literature. In addition, the choice between transcranial MEP surgeon-module and multimodal monitoring performed by a specialist was at the discretion of the chief surgeon. Most of the idiopathic scoliosis were flexible and of low magnitude, with a reducibility index of 2.22 on average (Cincinnati index). In our study, we had no cases of vertebral osteotomy or major scoliosis above 90° who may require complex surgery: two-stage surgery (anterior approach followed by posterior arthrodesis or halo gravity traction preparation or temporary internal distraction). Any such cases were operated under multimodal monitoring performed by a neurologist specialized in electrophysiology. Previous studies [11,12] using the transcranial MEP surgeon module have shown that it can be used in cases of complex deformities with safety and efficiency. In opposition, some authors show that a combined anterior/posterior approach has been associated with a significant increase in the risk of neurological lesion (OR, 0.23; 95% CI, 0.08 to 0.81; $p = 0.02$) [22]. With improved surgical techniques, two-stage surgery (anterior and posterior) is more prone to complications [23]. Several studies have demonstrated the effectiveness of IOM in vertebral resection surgery or in severe deformities [24,25]. But 41% of severe scoliosis (major cobb angle of 80 or more) showed intraoperative changes in SSEP neuromonitoring [26]. Based on our experience, we believe that is preferable to have a neurophysiologist present in complex deformities cases. Firstly, to obtain more reliable multimodal recordings that are less subject to anesthetic variation or homeostasis. Secondly, this allows the surgeon to concentrate on the complex surgical procedure itself [27]. Moreover, our mid-term clinical and radiographic follow-up was poorly reported. No quality-of-life scores were collected, and only the radiographic measurement of the post-operative Cobb angle was reported in Table 1. All patients were seen post-operatively (covering the period from day one to three months post-operatively) in line with the aim of the study, and only the analysis of the clinical examination during this period was reported in the results section.

Lastly, this study is a single-center study. The results might not be representative of other surgical centers, potentially limiting the external validity and applicability of the findings. This potential bias is mitigated by the large number of subjects included in our article, and that our results are similar to those of the other two prior studies [11,12] using different correction techniques (previously discussed).

5. Conclusions

Simplified transcranial MEP monitoring known as "surgeon-directed module" is usable, safe and reliable in surgery for moderate scoliosis after a learning curve. It is possible to achieve a reliable response in 95% of cases with at least four of the eight muscle sites tested and with a negative predictive value of 100%. Particular attention should be paid to cases of cerebral palsy where it is difficult to achieve a motor response of transcranial MEP. In such cases who require at least partially functional motor pathways, it may be worthwhile to schedule a preoperative consultation to analyze motor responses and confirm the feasibility of monitoring. Some neuromonitoring devices used by surgeons alone allow joint motor and somesthetic-evoked potentials, but their feasibility and training have yet to be evaluated, particularly in cases of severe deformity.

Author Contributions: Conceptualization, F.A. and A.K.; methodology, R.C.; software, P.H.; validation, J.S.d.G., F.A. and T.L.; formal analysis, T.L.; investigation, R.C.; resources, J.S.d.G.; data curation, P.H.; writing—original draft preparation, A.K.; writing—review and editing, T.L.; supervision, J.S.d.G. All authors have read and agreed to the published version of the manuscript.

Funding: This research received no external funding.

Institutional Review Board Statement: The study has been approved by a local ethics committee (IRB No. 22-03; approval date 15 February 2022). It was also registered in the National Committee of Computer Science and Liberties register (No. 22300620v0); once legal guardians of each patient were individually informed, charts review was conducted following the 1964 Declaration of Helsinki ethical standards and the Methodology of Reference MR-003.

Informed Consent Statement: Informed consent was obtained from all subjects involved in the study.

Data Availability Statement: The data presented in this study are available on request from the corresponding author. The data are not publicly available due to ethical restrictions.

Conflicts of Interest: The authors declare no conflict of interest.

References

1. Hamilton, D.K.; Smith, J.S.; Sansur, C.A.; Glassman, S.D.; Ames, C.P.; Berven, S.H.; Polly, D.W., Jr.; Perra, J.H.; Knapp, D.R.; Boachie-Adjei, O.; et al. Rates of new neurological deficit associated with spine surgery based on 108,419 procedures: A report of the scoliosis research society morbidity and mortality committee. *Spine* **2011**, *36*, 1218–1228. [CrossRef] [PubMed]
2. Kwan, K.Y.H.; Koh, H.Y.; Blanke, K.M.; Cheung, K.M.C. Complications following surgery for adolescent idiopathic scoliosis over a 13-year period. *Bone Jt. J.* **2020**, *102*, 519–523. [CrossRef] [PubMed]
3. Kwan, M.K.; Loh, K.W.; Chung, W.H.; Chiu, C.K.; Hasan, M.S.; Chan, C.Y.W. Perioperative outcome and complications following single-staged Posterior Spinal Fusion (PSF) using pedicle screw instrumentation in Adolescent Idiopathic Scoliosis (AIS): A review of 1057 cases from a single centre. *BMC Musculoskelet. Disord.* **2021**, *22*, 413. [CrossRef] [PubMed]
4. Weiss, H.-R.; Goodall, D. Rate of complications in scoliosis surgery—A systematic review of the Pub Med literature. *Scoliosis* **2008**, *3*, 9. [CrossRef] [PubMed]
5. Accadbled, F.; Henry, P.; de Gauzy, J.S.; Cahuzac, J.P. Spinal cord monitoring in scoliosis surgery using an epidural electrode. results of a prospective, consecutive series of 191 cases. *Spine* **2006**, *31*, 2614–2623. [CrossRef]
6. Scoliosis Research Society. *Scoliosis Research Society Position Statement. Somatosensory Evoked Potential Monitoring of Neurologic Spinal Cord Function during Spinal Surgery*; Scoliosis Research Society: Kansas City, MO, USA, 1992.
7. Gavaret, M.; Jouve, J.; Péréon, Y.; Accadbled, F.; André-Obadia, N.; Azabou, E.; Blondel, B.; Bollini, G.; Delécrin, J.; Farcy, J.-P.; et al. Intraoperative neurophysiologic monitoring in spine surgery. Developments and state of the art in France in 2011. *Orthop. Traumatol. Surg. Res.* **2013**, *99*, S319–S327. [CrossRef]
8. Merton, P.A.; Morton, H.B. Stimulation of the cerebral cortex in the intact human subject. *Nature* **1980**, *285*, 227. [CrossRef]
9. Ito, Z.; Matsuyama, Y.; Ando, M.; Kawabata, S.; Kanchiku, T.; Kida, K.; Fujiwara, Y.; Yamada, K.; Yamamoto, N.; Kobayashi, S.; et al. What is the best multimodality combination for intraoperative spinal cord monitoring of motor function? A multicenter study by the monitoring committee of the Japanese society for spine surgery and related research. *Glob. Spine J.* **2016**, *6*, 234–241. [CrossRef]
10. Pelosi, L.; Lamb, J.; Grevitt, M.; Mehdian, S.M.; Webb, J.K.; Blumhardt, L.D. Combined monitoring of motor and somatosensory evoked potentials in orthopaedic spinal surgery. *Clin. Neurophysiol.* **2002**, *113*, 1082–1091. [CrossRef]
11. Magampa, R.S.; Dunn, R. Surgeon-directed transcranial motor evoked potential spinal cord monitoring in spinal deformity surgery. *Bone Jt. J.* **2021**, *103*, 547–552. [CrossRef]
12. Chan, A.; Banerjee, P.; Lupu, C.; Bishop, T.; Bernard, J.; Lui, D. Surgeon-Directed Neuromonitoring in Adolescent Spinal Deformity Surgery Safely Assesses Neurological Function. *Cureus* **2021**, *13*, e19843. [CrossRef] [PubMed]
13. Langlais, T.; Rougereau, G.; Bruncottan, B.; Bolzinger, M.; Accadbled, F.; Compagnon, R.; Sales de Gauzy, J. Proximal Fixation in Adolescent Scoliosis Lenke 1 and 3 Treated by Posteromedial Translation Using Sublaminar Bands: Transverse-pedicular Hook Claw Versus Transverse Hook-pedicular Screw Claw. *Clin. Spine Surg.* **2021**, *34*, 377–382. [CrossRef] [PubMed]
14. Laumonerie, P.; Tibbo, M.E.; Kerezoudis, P.; Langlais, T.; de Gauzy, J.S.; Accadbled, F. Influence of the sublaminar band density in the treatment of Lenke 1 adolescent idiopathic scoliosis. *Orthop. Traumatol. Surg. Res.* **2020**, *106*, 1269–1274. [CrossRef] [PubMed]
15. Huss, G.K.; Betz, R.R.; Clancy, M. A draping technique for spinal surgery using the Stagnara wake-up test. *AORN J.* **1988**, *48*, 530–535. [CrossRef] [PubMed]

16. Noonan, K.J.; Walker, T.; Feinberg, J.R.; Nagel, M.; Didelot, W.; Lindseth, R. Factors related to false- versus true-positive neuromonitoring changes in adolescent idiopathic scoliosis surgery. *Spine* **2002**, *27*, 825–830. [CrossRef]
17. Shrader, M.W.; DiCindio, S.; Kenny, K.G.; Franco, A.J.; Zhang, R.; Theroux, M.C.; Rogers, K.J.; Shah, S.A. Transcranial electric motor evoked potential monitoring during scoliosis surgery in children with cerebral palsy and active seizure disorder: Is it feasible and safe? *Spine Deform.* **2023**; epub ahead of print.
18. Ushirozako, H.; Yoshida, G.; Hasegawa, T.; Yamato, Y.; Yasuda, T.; Banno, T.; Arima, H.; Oe, S.; Yamada, T.; Ide, K.; et al. Characteristics of false-positive alerts on transcranial motor evoked potential monitoring during pediatric scoliosis and adult spinal deformity surgery: An "anesthetic fade" phenomenon. *J. Neurosurg. Spine* **2019**, *32*, 423–431. [CrossRef]
19. Bhagat, S.; Durst, A.; Grover, H.; Blake, J.; Lutchman, L.; Rai, A.S.; Crawford, R. An evaluation of multimodal spinal cord monitoring in scoliosis surgery: A single centre experience of 354 operations. *Eur. Spine J.* **2015**, *24*, 1399–1407. [CrossRef]
20. Feng, B.; Qiu, G.; Shen, J.; Zhang, J.; Tian, Y.; Li, S.; Zhao, H.; Zhao, Y. Impact of multimodal intraoperative monitoring during surgery for spine deformity and potential risk factors for neurological monitoring changes. *J. Spinal Disord. Tech.* **2012**, *25*, E108–E114. [CrossRef]
21. Tsirikos, A.I.; Duckworth, A.D.; Henderson, L.E.; Michaelson, C. Multimodal Intraoperative Spinal Cord Monitoring during Spinal Deformity Surgery: Efficacy, Diagnostic Characteristics, and Algorithm Development. *Med. Princ. Pract.* **2019**, *29*, 6–17. [CrossRef]
22. Nassef, M.; Splinter, W.; Lidster, N.; Al-Kalbani, A.; Nashed, A.; Ilton, S.; Vanniyasingam, T.; Paul, J. Intraoperative neurophysiologic monitoring in idiopathic scoliosis surgery: A retrospective observational study of new neurologic deficits. *Can. J. Anaesth.* **2021**, *68*, 477–484. [CrossRef]
23. Hero, N.; Vengust, R.; Topolovec, M. Comparative Analysis of Combined (First Anterior, Then Posterior) Versus Only Posterior Approach for Treating Severe Scoliosis: A Mean Follow Up of 8.5 Years. *Spine* **2017**, *42*, 831–837. [CrossRef] [PubMed]
24. Skaggs, D.L.; Lee, C.; Myung, K.S. Neuromonitoring Changes Are Common and Reversible With Temporary Internal Distraction for Severe Scoliosis. *Spine Deform.* **2014**, *2*, 61–69. [CrossRef] [PubMed]
25. McClung, A.; Mundis, G.; Pawelek, J.; Garg, S.; Yaszay, B.; Boachie-Adjei, O.; James, O.S.; Sponseller, P.; Sánchez Pérez-Grueso, F.J.; Lavelle, W.; et al. Paper #19: Utilization and Reliability of Intraoperative Neuromonitoring in Vertebral Column Resections for Severe Early-Onset Scoliosis. *Spine Deform.* **2017**, *5*, 448–449.
26. MacDonald, D.B. Intraoperative motor evoked potential monitoring: Overview and update. *J. Clin. Monit. Comput.* **2006**, *20*, 347–377. [CrossRef]
27. Huang, Z.-F.; Chen, L.; Yang, J.-F.; Deng, Y.-L.; Sui, W.-Y.; Yang, J.-L. Multimodality Intraoperative Neuromonitoring in Severe Thoracic Deformity Posterior Vertebral Column Resection Correction. *World Neurosurg.* **2019**, *127*, e416–e426. [CrossRef] [PubMed]

Disclaimer/Publisher's Note: The statements, opinions and data contained in all publications are solely those of the individual author(s) and contributor(s) and not of MDPI and/or the editor(s). MDPI and/or the editor(s) disclaim responsibility for any injury to people or property resulting from any ideas, methods, instructions or products referred to in the content.

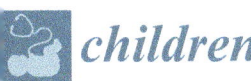

Article

Optimising Intraoperative Fluid Management in Patients Treated with Adolescent Idiopathic Scoliosis—A Novel Strategy for Improving Outcomes

Jakub Miegoń [1,*], Sławomir Zacha [2], Karolina Skonieczna-Żydecka [3], Agata Wiczk-Bratkowska [1], Agata Andrzejewska [1], Konrad Jarosz [4], Monika Deptuła-Jarosz [5] and Jowita Biernawska [1]

1. Department of Anaesthesiology and Intensive Care, Pomeranian Medical University in Szczecin, 71-252 Szczecin, Poland
2. Department of Paediatric Orthopaedics and Oncology of the Musculoskeletal System, Pomeranian Medical University in Szczecin, 71-252 Szczecin, Poland
3. Department of Biochemical Science, Pomeranian Medical University in Szczecin, 71-460 Szczecin, Poland
4. Department of Clinical Nursing, Pomeranian Medical University in Szczecin, 71-210 Szczecin, Poland
5. Department of Neurosurgery and Paediatric Neurosurgery, Pomeranian Medical University in Szczecin, 71-252 Szczecin, Poland
* Correspondence: jakub.miegon@gmail.com

Abstract: Scoliosis surgery is a challenge for the entire team in terms of safety, and its accomplishment requires the utilization of advanced monitoring technologies. A prospective, single centre, non-randomised controlled cohort study, was designed to assess the efficacy of protocolised intraoperative haemodynamic monitoring and goal-directed therapy in relation to patient outcomes following posterior fusion surgery for adolescent idiopathic scoliosis (AIS). The control group ($n = 35$, mean age: 15 years) received standard blood pressure management during the surgical procedure, whereas the intervention group ($n = 35$, mean age: 14 years) underwent minimally invasive haemodynamic monitoring. Arterial pulse contour analysis (APCO) devices were employed, along with goal-directed therapy protocol centered on achieving target mean arterial pressure and stroke volume. This was facilitated through the application of crystalloid boluses, ephedrine, and noradrenaline. The intervention group was subjected to a comprehensive protocol following Enhanced Recovery After Surgery (ERAS) principles. Remarkably, the intervention group exhibited notable advantages ($p < 0.05$), including reduced hospital stay durations (median 7 days vs. 10), shorter episodes of hypotension (mean arterial pressure < 60 mmHg—median 8 vs. 40 min), lesser declines in postoperative haemoglobin levels (−2.36 g/dl vs. −3.83 g/dl), and quicker extubation times. These compelling findings strongly imply that the integration of targeted interventions during the intraoperative care of AIS patients undergoing posterior fusion enhance a set of treatment outcomes.

Keywords: adolescent idiopathic scoliosis; haemodynamic monitoring; hypotension; length of stay; ERAS (enhanced recovery after surgery)

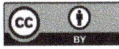

1. Introduction

Posterior fusion surgery for adolescent idiopathic scoliosis (AIS) poses a significant challenge to anaesthetists due to the extensive surgical area and the need for specific anaesthesia techniques that accommodate intraoperative neurophysiological monitoring of the spinal cord. AIS, the most common spinal deformity in children, necessitates surgical correction while minimising the risk of spinal cord injury, which can be achieved through intraoperative neuromonitoring and the maintenance of adequate spinal cord perfusion. In our centre, when qualifying for scoliosis, the criteria outlined in the Scoliosis Research Society (SRS) guidelines are followed, which means that scoliosis surgery is indicated for patients above 12 years of age with a Cobb angle > 45 degrees, without the necessity of general symptoms. For patients with early-onset scoliosis, two criteria must be met-both a Cobb angle > 45 degrees and a progression of more than 10 degrees per year [1]. The orthopaedics do not wait for complications in the form of organ dysfunction to arise. If the Cobb angle is less than 45 degrees, conservative treatment of scoliosis is possible. For angles below 30 degrees, rehabilitation is applied, and for angles above 30 degrees, bracing is considered, provided that the patient cooperates with this therapy.The maintenance of intraoperative haemodynamic stability holds significant importance in determining the postoperative prognosis of AIS patients undergoing surgical intervention. Hypotension, leading to tissue hypoperfusion, is a key contributor to unfavourable neurological outcomes. Monitoring parameters such as intraoperative volemia, cardiac function, blood pressure, and haemoglobin levels play a pivotal role in ensuring sufficient oxygen delivery to vital organs. Tissue hypoxia stands out as a major driver of perioperative complications [2]. Appropriate management of fluid administration and vasopressors becomes essential in preventing and treating hypo- and hypervolemia, while maintaining adequate oxygen delivery without causing fluid overload.

Intraoperative hypotension (IOH) frequently occurs during surgical procedures. However, a universally accepted definition for IOH remains elusive. IOH poses the potential for ischemia-reperfusion injury, which can manifest as dysfunction in vital organs [3]. While some studies have reported the association of IOH with postoperative complications in adults, similar investigations in children are scarce. The APRICOT study documented hypotension in 54.9% of major cardiovascular events, with the majority of these events (94%) resulting in uneventful outcomes [4].

Standard methods based on non-invasive blood pressure monitoring may not be sufficient to detect perfusion abnormalities. Hypovolemia can mask itself with normal blood pressure due to increased vascular resistance, and anaesthesia can influence heart rate, making it an unreliable indicator of hypovolemia. Moreover, oscillometric techniques, in comparison to invasive blood pressure measurement, tend to overestimate low blood pressure readings and underestimate high blood pressure readings. Consequently, more advanced haemodynamic monitoring methods have been developed.

Uncalibrated devices utilise patient anthropometric and demographic data, along with internal databases and algorithms, to calculate cardiac output (CO) from arterial waveforms, which proves valuable in perioperative optimisation protocols. Measured, calculated or derived haemodynamic parameters are instrumental in identifying the underlying causes of hypotension.

Goal-directed therapy (GDT) constitutes a haemodynamic treatment approach that involves titrating fluid and inotropic agents based on physiological flow-related endpoints [5]. Its implementation has shown to reduce perioperative morbidity and mortality in both adult and paediatric populations [6–13]. However, the application of monitoring methods primarily developed for adults to children may introduce challenges due to differing characteristics of the vascular system and the absence of reference values [14,15].

Paediatric patients exhibit a poor correlation between advanced haemodynamic parameters routinely used in adults, such as arterial pressure or plethysmographically derived variables, and fluid responsiveness [14]. This discrepancy in correlation with adults can be attributed to greater vascular compliance in paediatric patients. However, the precise age at which arterial properties in children resemble those in adults remains unknown, necessitating further research.

The objective of this study was to assess the effectiveness of a protocolised care approach involving intraoperative haemodynamic monitoring and goal-directed therapy in improving patient outcomes following posterior fusion surgery for AIS.

2. Materials and Methods

A prospective, single-centre, non-randomised, controlled cohort study was employed. The research focused on 70 consecutive Caucasian teenagers with AIS who underwent posterior fusion. The criteria for inclusion in the study were as follows: individuals who had their first scoliosis operation and were under 18 years of age. Patients who met the qualification for scoliosis surgery at this facility underwent X-ray imaging, computed tomography, and magnetic resonance imaging. Those with a Cobb angle exceeding 45 degrees were deemed eligible. Prior to anaesthesia approval, echocardiography and spirometry tests were conducted. Criteria used to exclude patients from the study included emergency surgery, reoperation, advanced chronic respiratory-circulatory failure, or scoliosis caused by factors other than idiopathic origins.

The control group, comprising of 35 patients with a mean age of 15 years, including 7 boys, received standard blood pressure management during the surgical procedure. Subsequently, the obtained results were analyzed to establish the protocol for the intervention group. The intervention group consisted of 35 patients, with a mean age of 14 years and a higher proportion of females (5 boys). This group followed a protocol that involved intraoperative minimally invasive haemodynamic monitoring, GDT, and components of Enhanced Recovery After Surgery (ERAS). The study's participant flow is visually represented in Figure 1 using the Consort diagram.

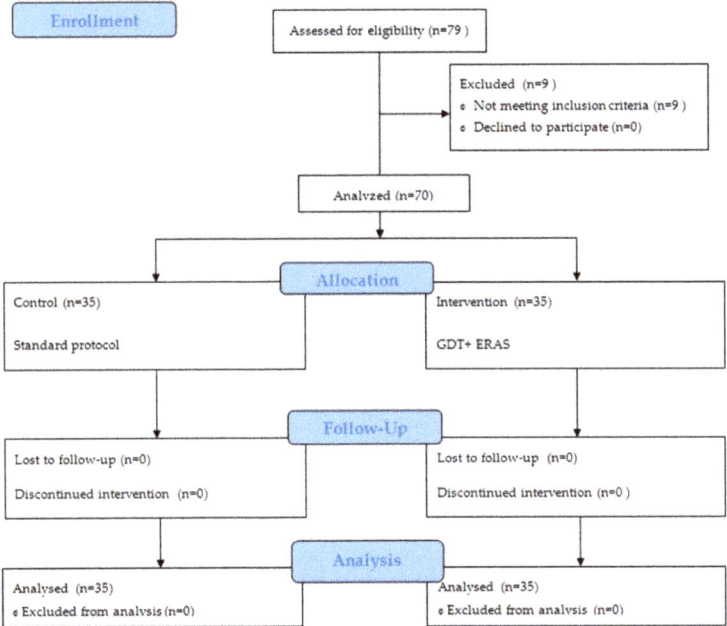

Figure 1. The Consort diagram.

The study protocol was officially registered with the clinicaltrials.gov database and can be identified by the accession number NCT 05159505.

2.1. Preparation for Surgery

In preparation for the scheduled surgery, patients were directed to undergo an anaesthetic consultation and subsequently were qualified for general anaesthesia.

On the day of the operation, as a pre-emptive analgesia, patients were administered metamizole at a dosage of 15 mg/kg for children weighing under 50 kg, or a 1 g oral dose if body weight exceeded 50 kg. Additionally, they received an orally administered carbohydrate-rich fluid (Preop, Nutricia, Poland).

2.2. Surgery

During the procedure, all patients received general anaesthesia, which involved intubation using a reinforced endotracheal tube and mechanical ventilation using a Primus apparatus (Dräger, Germany). The control group did not adhere to a specific anaesthesia protocol, as the decision regarding analgesic medications and anaesthesia management was left to the administering anaesthesiologist. A visual representation of the anaesthesia administration in the intervention group can be found in Figure 2. In this group, patients had a radial artery catheter placed for arterial access, and an HemoSphere (Edwards Lifesciences, Irvine, CA, USA) monitor and a Flotrac or Acumen IQ sensor was utilised for haemodynamic monitoring purposes.

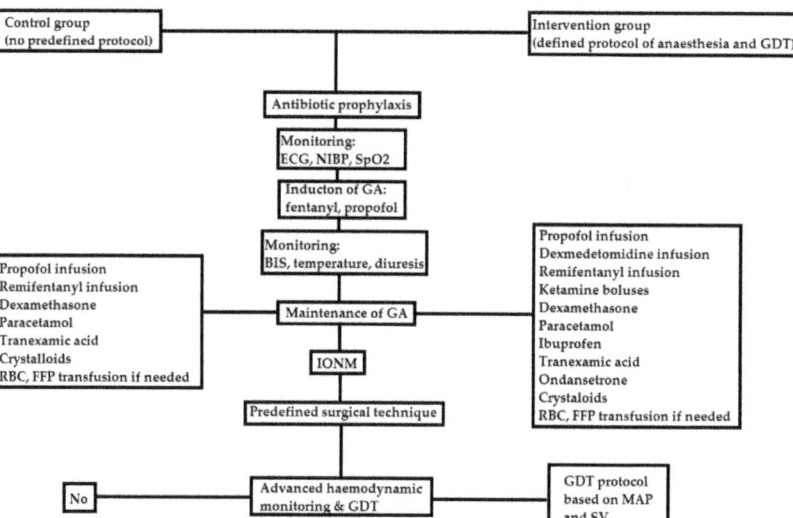

Figure 2. The anaesthesia protocol used in this study (ECG—electrocardiography, NIBP—non-invasive blood pressure, SpO2—pulse oximetry, GA—general anaesthesia, RBC—red blood cells, FFP—fresh frozen plasma, IONM—intraoperative neuromonitoring, GDT—goal directed therapy, MAP—mean arterial pressure, SV—stroke volume).

In this study, a GDT protocol was implemented, aiming to maintain the desired levels of mean arterial pressure (MAP) and stroke volume (SV) by means of fluid therapy and the administration of vasopressors. A detailed outline of the protocol can be found in Figure 3.

Fluid therapy in this study encompassed the administration of balanced crystalloid solutions (Sterofundin-B. Braun/Optilyte-Fresenius Kabi) intravenously at a rate of 4:2:1 mL/kg/h. The initiation of the protocol occurred when the patient was transitioned to the prone position, preceded by an intravenous bolus of 5 mg ephedrine to address hypotension. The target values aimed to maintain MAP above 60 mmHg, with a higher threshold of MAP > 75 mmHg in cases of depressed MEP.

If hypotension (MAP < 60 mmHg) and SV below 50 mL/beat were observed, a crystalloid bolus of 5 mL/kg was administered intravenously over a period of 10–15 min. Following the bolus, the response to fluid therapy was evaluated. If SV increased by more than 10% and hypotension persisted, an additional fluid bolus was given. In cases where SV did not increase by more than 10%, norepinephrine infusion was initiated to sustain a MAP above 60 mmHg.

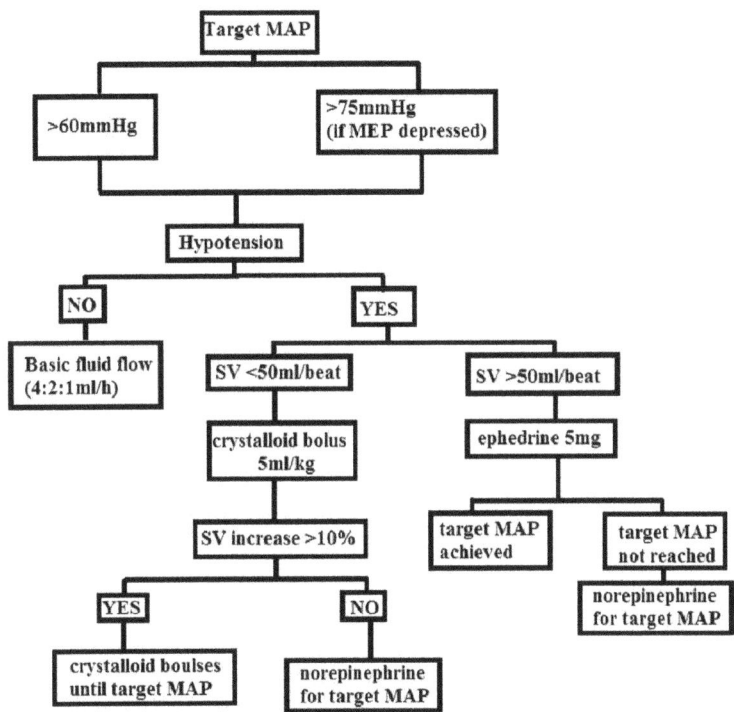

Figure 3. The GDT protocol used in this study, adapted from Edwards Lifesciences protocol [16] (MAP—mean arterial pressure, MEP—motor-evoked potentials, SV—stroke volume).

When hypotension (MAP < 60 mmHg) was present but SV exceeded 50 ml/beat, a single dose of 5 mg ephedrine was administered. If the response was insufficient, norepinephrine infusion was initiated to maintain the target MAP. In situations where SV was below 50 mL/beat but no evidence of hypotension (MAP > 60 mmHg) or peripheral perfusion failure (capillary refill time < 2 s) was observed, no fluid bolus was administered. The use of colloids for fluid administration was prohibited. In cases where blood loss surpassed 7 mL/kg, a transfusion of 1 unit of red blood cells was provided.

The extubation criteria were not firmly defined in the study. They considered the presence of spontaneous breathing, the level of consciousness-responsiveness to voice with eye opening, the presence of gag reflex, and hemodynamic stability.

2.3. Surgical Technique

The surgical procedure employed a posterior approach, involving ligament and bone release, implant fixations, and the ultimate correction using titanium rods. The surgical techniques utilised either a screws-only system or hybrid systems incorporating screws, hooks, or sublaminar bands.

2.4. Intraoperative Neuromonitoring (IONM)

Continuous monitoring of motor and sensory potentials was carried out throughout the procedure to ensure the preservation of spinal cord function. The IONM was performed using the Inomed Neurstimulator ISIS device, following a consistent protocol. The placement of screws relative to the spinal root was verified using direct nerve stimulation (DNS) electromyography. DNS was conducted with a constant current (CC) of 3 Hz frequency, 200 μs pulse duration, monopolar/negative stimulation, and a stimulation threshold of 8 mA. Additionally, the integrity of the corticospinal pathway was assessed during the correction procedure using transcranial electrostimulation (TES) or motor evoked potentials (MEP). TES/MEP involved CC with 2 Hz frequency, interstimulus interval (ISI) of 4 mA, a train of 5 pulses, positive polarity, 500 µs pulse duration, and a maximum amplitude of 200 mA. The motor responses were recorded from indicator muscles of the lower extremities and upper extremity flexors, serving as a reference. Furthermore, somatosensory evoked potentials (SEP) were evaluated by stimulating the posterior tibial nerves with CC, square pulses/positive polarity, 200 µs pulse duration, 3.7 Hz frequency, and an amplitude of 25 mA, as an assessment of sensory pathway integrity.

2.5. Postoperative Course

Patients were monitored in the post-anaesthesia care unit (PACU) for a duration of 24 h after surgery. Vital signs were regularly assessed, and a numerical scale (NRS) was utilised to evaluate pain intensity. This assessment was performed every hour for the initial 24 h and then every 8 h until hospital discharge. The evaluation included monitoring the administered drugs, their type, dose, route, and any occurrence of side effects or complications.

During the postoperative period, medications such as paracetamol, metamizole, ibuprofen, magnesium sulfate, intravenous opioid infusion, and lide infusions were administered at regular intervals. The decision to transition from intravenous to oral treatment was determined based on the patient's daily requirements.

The study maintained consistency in preoperative preparation, surgical technique, perioperative analgesia, and postoperative evaluation parameters between the "control" and "intervention" groups. The intervention group followed a hospitalisation plan rooted in the principles of the ERAS protocol. ERAS programs employ a multidisciplinary approach to improve surgical outcomes by implementing evidence-based, procedure-specific care protocols. In this study, the ERAS program encompassed elements such as early mobilisation, rehabilitation, early evacuation of drains, early initiation of oral hydration, and early initiation of feeding.

2.6. Definitions of Complications

The evaluation of the obtained results was a comparison in terms of: demographic data, total time of hypotension, duration of the surgical procedure "skin to skin" (minutes), duration of hospitalisation (days).

Hypotension in the study was defined as systolic blood pressure (SBP) below 90 mmHg and MAP below 60 mmHg for at least 1 min. Adverse drug reactions encompassed symptoms such as apnoea, dyspnoea, decrease in SpO2 below 90%, bradycardia, hypotension, pruritus, nausea, vomiting, urinary retention, constipation, dizziness and drowsiness preventing rehabilitation. Surgical complications included partial or complete spinal cord injury leading to transient or persistent paralysis, transient neuropraxia related to positioning, dural tear, position-related complications, visual disturbances, respiratory-circulatory failure, surgical site infection, haematoma, gastric disorders, pneumonia, and death. In order to assess the findings, a comparative analysis was conducted, which involved examining demographic data, total duration of hypotension, the length of the surgical procedure from "skin to skin" in minutes, and the duration of hospitalisation in days.

2.7. Outcomes

The primary outcome of the study was the duration of hospitalisation in days. Additionally, secondary outcomes were evaluated, including the following: intraoperative hypotension time (min), volume of red blood cell transfusion (mL), volume of fresh frozen plasma transfusion (mL), intraoperative blood loss (mL), administration of crystalloids (mL/kg), total dose of ephedrine (mg), pre-surgery haemoglobin level (g/dL), post-surgery haemoglobin level (g/dL), change in haemoglobin level (g/dL), pre-surgery haematocrit level (%), post-surgery haematocrit level (%), change in haematocrit level (%),the duration of the surgical procedure "skin to skin" (min), and time to extubation (min), the occurrence of neurological and cardiac complications.

2.8. Statistical Analyses

To assess the distribution of continuous variables, the Shapiro-Wilk normality test was conducted. Descriptive statistics were then reported using means and standard deviations, or median and interquartile ranges (IQR), as appropriate. Qualitative variables were presented as numbers and percentages. For comparing outcomes between the two groups, either the nonparametric Mann-Whitney test or parametric t-test was employed. The chi-squared test was utilised to analyze the association between qualitative variables. For the variables with low numbers ($n < 5$), a Fisher's exact test was adopted. The significance level for type I error was set at 0.05, and the calculations were performed using MedCalc statistical software version 20.110 (Ostend, Belgium). To control for type I errors, the false discovery rate (FDR) approach was applied using the p.adjust function from the stats package in R [17]. The statistical power was determined using G*Power software version 3.1.9.2 [18].

3. Results

3.1. Study Participants

Table 1 presents the baseline characteristics of the study participants in relation to the tested procedure. No statistically significant differences were observed among any of the tested parameters except of haemoglobin level. Patients within the control group had a higher concentration as compared to intervention group counterparts.

Table 1. Demographic data from patients among the groups.

Parameters	Control ($n = 35$)	Intervention ($n = 35$)	p
Age	15 (14–17) *	14 (13–17) *	0.144
Gender (boys/girls)	7/28	5/30	0.529
BMI	20.58 (18.43–22.36) *	18.97 (17.93–21.77) *	0.259
Haemoglobin level before surgery (g/dL)	13.71 (1.326) **	13.03 (0.93) *	0.016
Haematocrit level before surgery (%)	38.29 (4.03) **	37.93 (2.72) **	0.672
ASA * 1	21	22	0.297
ASA 2	14	10	
ASA >2	0	3	

Legend: BMI—body mass index, ASA—American Society of Anaesthesiology; * median, interquartile range; ** mean, standard deviation.

3.2. Outcomes

Table 2 presents a comprehensive comparison of perioperative data, hypotension time, complications, transfusions, and haemoglobin levels between the control and intervention groups. The results demonstrate that intraoperative haemodynamic monitoring had a significant impact on various outcomes, including duration of hospital stay, number of neurological and cardiac complications, hypotension time, fresh frozen plasma (FFP) transfusion, time to extubation, and all tested blood parameters. Notably, the intervention group exhibited minimal duration of hypotension with MAP below 55 mmHg, with a median of 0 min and an interquartile range (IQR) of 0–3.5 min. The intervention group did not require the administration of norepinephrine throughout the study.

Table 2. Perioperative data, time of hypotension, complications, transfusions.

Parameters	Control (n = 35)	Intervention (n = 35)	p	FDR	Power
Duration of the surgical procedure "skin to skin" (minutes)	195 (16–218) *	205 (170–240) *	0.390	0.442	0.52
Neurological complications (no)	1	0	0.5	0.531	0.32
Cardiac complications (no)	3	0	0.239	0.290	0.66
Duration of hospitalisation (days)	10 (9–11) *	7 (6–8) *	<0.001	0.003	0.99
Hypotension time (min)	40 (20–60) *	8 (1–14) *	<0.001	0.003	0.98
Red blood cells transfusion volume (mL)	290 (0–560) *	190 (0–290) *	0.123	0.16	0.48
Fresh frozen plasma transfusion volume (mL)	200 (0–200) *	0 *	<0.001	0.003	0.99
Intraoperative blood loss (mL)	500 (350–500) *	500 (350–588) *	0.903	0.903	0.07
Crystalloids administered (mL/kg)	22 (16.3–31.5) *	27.8 (20.1–35.4) *	0.078	0.121	0.4
Ephedrine total dose (mg)	0 (0–8.75) *	5 (0–13.75) *	0.098	0.139	0.05
Intraoperative fluid administration (mL)	23.5 (10.05)	27.8 (9.93)	0.078	0.121	0.4
Haemoglobin level after surgery (g/dL)	9.71 (1.59) **	10.67 (1.02) **	0.007	0.017	0.74
Change in haemoglobin ^ (g/dL)	−3.83 (1.50) **	−2.36 (1.14) **	<0.001	0.006	0.97
Haematocrit level after surgery (%)	27.93 (4.05) **	31.05 (3.18) **	0.002	0.064	0.87
Change in haematocrit level ^ (%)	−9.53 (5.39) **	−6.89 (3.69) **	0.030	0.003	0.53
Time to extubation $ (min)	27.5 (20–50) *	0 (0–15) *	<0.001	0.115	0.99
Intraoperative diuresis (mL)	135 (100–250)	215 (127–300)	0.061	0.442	0.21

Legend: * median, interquartile range; ** mean, SD; ^ before-after surgery; $ time from end of operation till extubation.

Exemplary Figures 4 and 5 of significant results are presented below.

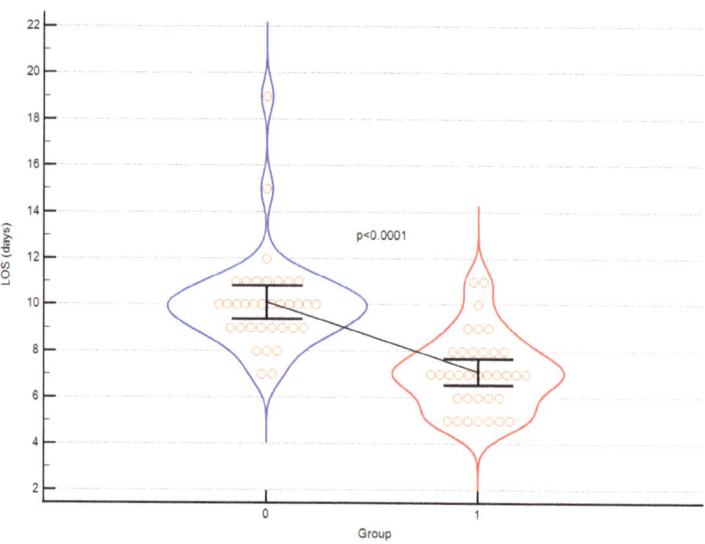

Figure 4. A violin plot depicting the length of hospital stay between control (0) and intervention (1) group. Orange circles represent individual cases. The black horizontal line connects means. Error bars represent SD.

In the control group, exclusively, four complications of neurological and cardiac nature were observed (cardiorespiratory failure resulting from hypovolemic shock—three patients, transient limb paresis—one patient). None of these events occurred among the subjects in the intervention group. It is noteworthy to mention that the hypovolemic shock in the control group was due to a gradual rather than sudden blood loss, which eventually proved to be significant and life-threatening. Consequently, these patients required postoperative intensive care, and one of them additionally developed a complication in the form of pneumonia. Unfortunately, we were not able to assess by means of statistics whether the complications occur less frequently when an invasive haemodynamic monitoring is introduced, as no such data were obtained in the intervention group. More studies to verify these results are warranted.

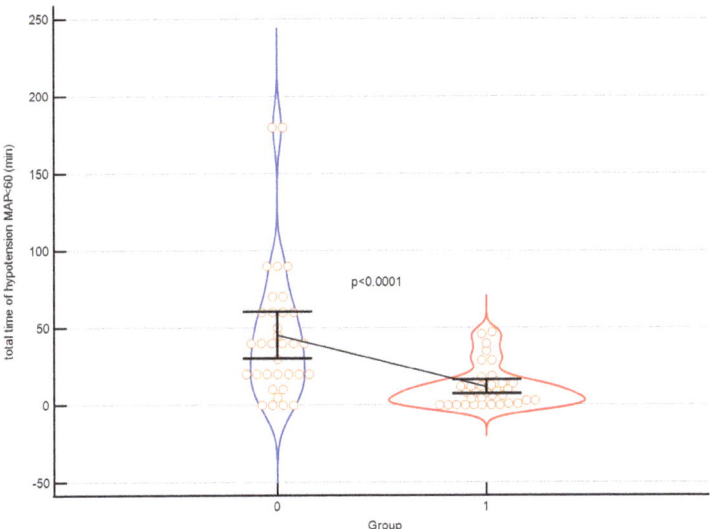

Figure 5. A violin plot depicting the perioperative hypotension time between control (0) and intervention (1) group. Orange circles represent individual cases. The black horizontal line connects medians. Error bars represent IQRs.

4. Discussion

This study aimed to assess the efficacy of intraoperative haemodynamic monitoring GDT outcomes in adolescents undergoing posterior fusion for AIS.

Firstly, the intervention group demonstrated a significantly shorter length of stay in hospital. Furthermore, patients in the intervention group displayed a substantially reduced duration of hypotension (MAP < 60 mmHg). Additionally, it is worth mentioning that the intraoperative diuresis was higher in the control group, while the GDT approach resulted in more stable haemoglobin and haematocrit levels with a smaller amplitude of changes and improved blood pressure stability. The extent of blood loss remained similar in both groups, albeit FFP was more frequently transfused in the control group. Additionally, the time interval from the conclusion of surgery to extubation was notably shorter in the intervention group, which contributed to earlier patient mobilisation. The duration of surgical procedures did not exhibit any notable differences between the two groups, which can be attributed to the consistent involvement of the same surgical team. Remarkably, the control group experienced instances of cardiac and neurological complications, whereas no such adverse events were observed in the intervention group following the implementation of the GDT protocol. These findings emphasise the potential of the intervention to enhance post-operative recovery and overall patient outcomes. The results obtained by the authors were corrected for multiple testing and statistical power was calculated for each comparison to demonstrate the validity. As elegantly summarised in Table 2, the following outcomes gained high statistical power: duration of hospitalisation, hypotension time, FFP transfusion volume, change in haemoglobin, time to extubation. Also, in regard to these results, the differences between intervention group and control group remained statistically significant after multiple testing. The authors hereby confirm, that invasive haemodynamic monitoring in teenagers with AIS is efficient with respect to many of intra and postoperative parameters

The observed reduction in length of stay within our study can be attributed to a range of factors, with particular emphasis on the absence of complications within the intervention group and the successful implementation of the ERAS strategy for uncomplicated patients. A study conducted by Marsollier et al., which harnessed the ERAS protocol for AIS cases, demonstrated a noteworthy decrease in the median length of hospital stay within the ERAS group [19]. Additionally, research by Jeandel et al., focusing on ERAS utilization for AIS, showcased not only a decrease in hospital stay but also a significant reduction in hospitalization costs [20]. These findings collectively underscore the significance of the ERAS approach in optimizing postoperative outcomes and resource utilization in AIS cases.

According to surveys conducted by the Scoliosis Research Society, spinal deformity surgery carries a risk of spinal cord injury, with reported rates ranging from 0.3% to 0.6% [21]. These injuries to the spinal cord can arise from various factors, including direct compression by surgical instruments or implants, compromised blood flow due to vessel stretching or compression, interruption of radicular blood flow, spinal cord distraction injury, or the presence of epidural haematoma. Among these factors, ischemic injury is the most commonly observed, with the motor pathways supplied by the anterior spinal artery being particularly susceptible to such damage. Therefore, timely identification and prevention of hypotension during spinal deformity surgery are vital in reducing the risk of ischemic injury. However, detecting hypotension early can pose challenges, especially in paediatric patients, due to the limited availability of non-invasive monitoring options.

To address the aforementioned challenges, the utilisation of invasive monitoring and GDT emerges as a potential solution, given its proven advantages in adult populations. Hence, the objective of this study is to assess the potential advantages of GDT in minimizing the duration of hypotension episodes during scoliosis surgery, specifically focusing on the prevention of intraoperative spinal cord ischemia, which is recognised as the most prevalent complication.

The selection of a MAP threshold of less than 60 mmHg as an indicator of hypotension in this study was driven by several considerations. Notably, there are no established hypotension thresholds specific to the age group of teenagers undergoing spinal deformity surgery. Given that the study population consisted of slim teenagers who likely possessed good microcirculation autoregulation, the authors believed that a lower threshold would be appropriate for detecting deviations from normal blood pressure ranges. Additionally, previous research has demonstrated that maintaining a MAP above 60 mm Hg during spinal surgery is a critical factor in lowering the likelihood of spinal cord injury, aligning with the observations made by the authors [22]. This evidence supports the notion that maintaining an adequate perfusion pressure is crucial for safeguarding the integrity of the spinal cord. By selecting a MAP threshold of less than 60 mmHg, the authors aimed to establish a clinically relevant cut-off that would prompt timely intervention to prevent hypotension-related complications. This threshold takes into account the unique characteristics of the study population while aligning with the existing literature on the importance of maintaining appropriate blood pressure levels during spinal surgery. While the Flotrac APCO system has demonstrated utility in the paediatric population, it is important to note that its validation specifically in children is yet to be established.

The findings of this study demonstrate that the combination of invasive arterial pressure monitoring and the implementation of the GDT protocol leads to a significant reduction in the duration of intraoperative hypotension. Notably, it was observed that the instances where the MAP remained below 55 mmHg were remarkably transient, indicating effective management of blood pressure during the surgical procedure.

GDT protocols have gained significant popularity in the operating theatre as a means to optimise the patient's haemodynamic status and enhance overall outcomes. Various types of GDT protocols can be employed, such as those focusing on CO, SV, and oxygen delivery optimisation. These protocols utilise advanced monitoring techniques, including arterial waveform analysis, pulse contour analysis, and echocardiography, to guide the administration of fluids and vasopressors with the aim of achieving specific haemodynamic targets. Alternatively, some protocols utilise dynamic variables like stroke volume variation (SVV) or pulse pressure variation (PPV) to guide fluid management decisions. The implementation of GDT has demonstrated notable improvements in outcomes across a range of surgical procedures, encompassing high-risk surgeries and major abdominal surgeries. The updated guidelines from the European Society of Cardiology (ESC) on cardiovascular assessment and management of patients undergoing non-cardiac surgery have assigned a Class IA recommendation for perioperative goal-directed haemodynamic therapy in high-risk surgical adult patients. Additionally, there is a strong recommendation (IB) to prevent an intraoperative decrease in MAP exceeding 20% from baseline or falling below the range of 60–70 mmHg to mitigate the occurrence of perioperative complications [23].

The use of GDT protocols has been extensively studied and implemented in the adult population; however, there is a scarcity of literature regarding their application in paediatric patients. A study conducted by Pereira de Souza Neto et al. focused on mechanically ventilated children under general anaesthesia, investigating the predictive value of dynamic parameters and transthoracic echocardiography in assessing fluid responsiveness [14]. The study findings indicated that while the respiratory variation of aortic peak velocity (ΔVpeak) proved to be an accurate predictor of fluid responsiveness, no arterial pressure or plethysmographically derived variable demonstrated accuracy in predicting fluid responsiveness.

On the other hand, Koraki et al. conducted a single-centre retrospective analysis utilising a GDT protocol based on SVV and ClearSight technology (Edwards Lifesciences) in scoliosis surgery [13]. The authors observed that this SVV and ClearSight-based GDT protocol effectively maintained haemodynamic stability and yielded favorable outcomes in patients undergoing scoliosis surgery. Notably, the protocol was associated with reduced requirements for blood transfusions, shorter hospital stays, and lower rates of postoperative complications. The results of these studies indicate the potential benefits of implementing GDT protocols in paediatric populations undergoing high-risk surgery, such as scoliosis correction. However, further research is necessary to determine the optimal approach to GDT in children and identify the most suitable protocols to improve outcomes within this specific population.

The choice of utilising an arterial waveform analysis GDT protocol, as opposed to pulse contour analysis or ultrasound analysis, is guided by multiple considerations. Firstly, arterial waveform analysis is a well-established and validated method that effectively evaluates fluid responsiveness, providing continuous and real-time feedback regarding haemodynamic fluctuations. In contrast, echocardiographic analysis necessitates specialised training and may not be feasible in all clinical settings. Furthermore, it is typically performed at specific time points and may not promptly detect acute changes in haemodynamic status. Non-invasive pulse contour analysis, on the other hand, may encounter challenges affected by factors such as hypothermia, vasoconstriction, or centralisation of circulation, ultimately compromising the accuracy of the technique.

In light of these factors, the authors have chosen to implement a GDT protocol based on SV. Alternative SVV-based protocols can pose challenges in clinical scenarios where there are variations in intra-thoracic pressure, such as during scoliosis correction. This is because SVV can be influenced by alterations in venous return and compliance, potentially leading to misinterpretation and inappropriate decisions regarding fluid management. Another aspect considered is that protocols relying on CO are more susceptible to variability due to fluctuations in heart rate, which can result in imprecise measurements, thus rendering them less dependable.

It is of utmost importance to acknowledge that during scoliosis correction procedures, the anaesthesiologist should exercise caution when implementing the conventional GDT protocol and remain mindful of its limitations in this specific surgical context. This is primarily due to instances where the surgeon exerts significant force, resulting in thoracic compression and potential kinking of the arterial cannula. Consequently, the arterial pressure waveform may exhibit a straight line pattern, which can be misinterpreted as hypotension. This ambiguity arises as the usual response to hypotension would involve initiating the GDT protocol. However, in the case of scoliosis correction procedures, it is crucial to recognise that the appropriate course of action is to adjust the force exerted by the surgeon on the surgical instruments. By appropriately modifying the applied force, it becomes possible to prevent hypotension and maintain optimal haemodynamic stability in the patient. Without clinician awareness of the importance of hypotension prevention and immediate treatment, the protocol will fail. Education and confidence in new tools is a very important part of success in hypotension prevention.

This study, despite its promising findings, is subject to several limitations that need to be acknowledged. Firstly, the study design employed was a non-randomised, single-centre, prospective, controlled cohort study, potentially restricting the generalisability of the results. The absence of randomization and the inclusion of patients solely from a single centre introduce the possibility of selection bias, thus not accurately representing the broader population of patients undergoing posterior fusion for adolescent idiopathic scoliosis. Additionally, the lack of blinding in the intervention group introduces the potential for performance bias since clinicians were aware of the treatment being administered.

Notwithstanding these limitations, this study offers valuable information regarding the potential advantages of intraoperative haemodynamic monitoring and GDT in patients with AIS. However, further exploration through larger, multicentre, randomised controlled trials is warranted to gain deeper insights and establish a more comprehensive understanding of the subject matter.

In summary, fluid management and protocolised haemodynamic monitoring have become integral elements of the paediatric ERAS (Enhanced Recovery After Surgery) protocol, offering significant potential benefits. When combined with intraoperative neuromonitoring, this approach holds promise in reducing hospital stays and minimising postoperative complications such as blood loss, neurological injuries, and wound infections. Recent studies have demonstrated that the implementation of haemodynamic optimisation and ERAS protocols can lead to improved outcomes, particularly in high-risk surgical procedures like scoliosis surgery. By employing real-time haemodynamic monitoring and goal-directed therapy protocols, healthcare providers can deliver personalised care tailored to individual patients' physiological requirements.

As ongoing research in this field progresses, it remains crucial to continually evaluate and compare different haemodynamic monitoring and fluid management protocols. This evaluation aims to identify the most effective approaches for enhancing outcomes and minimising complications in paediatric surgical patients. Further studies are warranted to refine protocols and establish best practice guidelines specifically for scoliosis surgery.

5. Conclusions

To summarise, the utilisation of intraoperative haemodynamic monitoring and goal-directed therapy in patients undergoing posterior fusion for AIS has demonstrated several positive outcomes. These include reduced hospital stay duration, shorter intraoperative hypotension time, and improved preservation of haemoglobin and haematocrit levels.

Author Contributions: Conceptualization, J.M., J.B., A.A. and K.J.; methodology, J.M., A.A., J.B., K.J. and M.D.-J.; validation, J.M.; formal analysis, K.S.-Ż.; investigation, J.M., S.Z., A.A., K.S.-Ż., K.J., A.W.-B. and J.B.; resources, S.Z.; data curation, J.M., S.Z., K.S.-Ż., K.J., A.W.-B., A.A. and J.B.; writing—original draft preparation, J.M. and A.A.; writing—review and editing, J.B. and S.Z.; visualization, J.M. and K.S.-Ż.; supervision, J.B.; project administration, J.B. All authors have read and agreed to the published version of the manuscript.

Funding: This research received no external funding.

Institutional Review Board Statement: The study was conducted in accordance with the Declaration of Helsinki, and approved by the Institutional Review Board at Pomeranian Medical University in Szczecin (resolution no. KB 0012/126/10/2021/Z; 27 October 2021).

Informed Consent Statement: All study participants over 16 years of age and their legal guardians gave informed consent to participate in the study, and participants under 16 years of age had informed consent obtained solely from their legal guardians. Written informed consent has been obtained from the patient(s) to publish this paper.

Data Availability Statement: The raw data are available upon request from the corresponding author.

Conflicts of Interest: The authors declare no conflict of interest.

References

1. Negrini, S.; Donzelli, S.; Aulisa, A.G.; Czaprowski, D.; Schreiber, S.; De Mauroy, J.C.; Diers, H.; Grivas, T.B.; Knott, P.; Kotwicki, T.; et al. 2016 SOSORT guidelines: Orthopaedic and rehabilitation treatment of idiopathic scoliosis during growth. *Scoliosis Spinal Disord.* **2018**, *13*, 3. [CrossRef]
2. Vincent, J.-L.; Pelosi, P.; Pearse, R.; Payen, D.; Perel, A.; Hoeft, A.; Romagnoli, S.; Ranieri, V.M.; Ichai, C.; Forget, P.; et al. Perioperative cardiovascular monitoring of high-risk patients: A consensus of 12. *Crit. Care* **2015**, *19*, 224. [CrossRef]
3. Walsh, M.; Devereaux, P.J.; Garg, A.X.; Kurz, A.; Turan, A.; Rodseth, R.N.; Cywinski, J.; Thabane, L.; Sessler, D.I. Relationship between Intraoperative Mean Arterial Pressure and Clinical Outcomes after Noncardiac Surgery: Toward an empirical definition of hypotension. *Anesthesiology* **2013**, *119*, 507–515. [CrossRef]
4. Habre, W.; Disma, N.; Virág, K.; Becke, K.; Hansen, T.G.; Jöhr, M.; Leva, B.; Morton, N.S.; Vermeulen, P.M.; Zielinska, M.; et al. Incidence of severe critical events in paediatric anaesthesia (APRICOT): A prospective multicentre observational study in 261 hospitals in Europe. *Lancet Respir. Med.* **2017**, *5*, 412–425. [CrossRef]
5. Dalfino, L.; Giglio, M.T.; Puntillo, F.; Marucci, M.; Brienza, N. Haemodynamic goal-directed therapy and postoperative infections: Earlier is better. a systematic review and meta-analysis. *Crit. Care* **2011**, *15*, R154. [CrossRef] [PubMed]
6. Rollins, K.E.; Lobo, D.N. Intraoperative Goal-directed Fluid Therapy in Elective Major Abdominal Surgery: A Meta-analysis of Randomized Controlled Trials. *Ann. Surg.* **2016**, *263*, 465–476. [CrossRef] [PubMed]
7. Bacchin, M.R.; Ceria, C.M.; Giannone, S.; Ghisi, D.; Stagni, G.; Greggi, T.; Bonarelli, S. Goal-Directed Fluid Therapy Based on Stroke Volume Variation in Patients Undergoing Major Spine Surgery in the Prone Position: A Cohort Study. *Spine* **2016**, *41*, E1131–E1137. [CrossRef] [PubMed]
8. Habicher, M.; Balzer, F.; Mezger, V.; Niclas, J.; Müller, M.; Perka, C.; Krämer, M.; Sander, M. Implementation of goal-directed fluid therapy during hip revision arthroplasty: A matched cohort study. *Perioper. Med.* **2016**, *5*, 31. [CrossRef] [PubMed]
9. Ripollés, J.; Espinosa, A.; Martínez-Hurtado, E.; Abad-Gurumeta, A.; Casans-Francés, R.; Fernández-Pérez, C.; López-Timoneda, F.; Calvo-Vecino, J.M. Intraoperative goal directed hemodynamic therapy in noncardiac surgery: A systematic review and meta-analysis. *Braz. J. Anesthesiol.* **2016**, *66*, 513–528. [CrossRef]
10. Dushianthan, A.; Knight, M.; Russell, P.; Grocott, M.P. Goal-directed haemodynamic therapy (GDHT) in surgical patients: Systematic review and meta-analysis of the impact of GDHT on post-operative pulmonary complications. *Perioper. Med.* **2020**, *9*, 30. [CrossRef]
11. Michard, F.; Giglio, M.T.; Brienza, N. Perioperative goal-directed therapy with uncalibrated pulse contour methods: Impact on fluid management and postoperative outcome. *Br. J. Anaesth.* **2017**, *119*, 22–30. [CrossRef] [PubMed]
12. Benes, J.; Giglio, M.; Brienza, N.; Michard, F. The effects of goal-directed fluid therapy based on dynamic parameters on post-surgical outcome: A meta-analysis of randomized controlled trials. *Crit. Care* **2014**, *18*, 584. [CrossRef] [PubMed]
13. Koraki, E.; Stachtari, C.; Stergiouda, Z.; Stamatopoulou, M.; Gkiouliava, A.; Sifaki, F.; Chatzopoulos, S.; Trikoupi, A. Blood and fluid management during scoliosis surgery: A single-center retrospective analysis. *Eur. J. Orthop. Surg. Traumatol.* **2020**, *30*, 809–814. [CrossRef]
14. Neto, E.P.d.S.; Grousson, S.; Duflo, F.; Ducreux, C.; Joly, H.; Convert, J.; Mottolese, C.; Dailler, F.; Cannesson, M. Predicting fluid responsiveness in mechanically ventilated children under general anaesthesia using dynamic parameters and transthoracic echocardiography. *Br. J. Anaesth.* **2011**, *106*, 856–864. [CrossRef]
15. De Graaff, J.C.; Pasma, W.; van Buuren, S.; Duijghuisen, J.J.; Nafiu, O.O.; Kheterpal, S.; van Klei, W.A. Reference Values for Noninvasive Blood Pressure in Children during Anesthesia: A Multicentered Retrospective Observational Cohort Study. *Anesthesiology* **2016**, *125*, 904–913. [CrossRef]
16. Edwards' Hemodynamic Optimization Reference Card. Irvine, USA. Available online: https://education.edwards.com/hemodynamic-optimization-reference-card/330963#hemosphere (accessed on 1 July 2023).
17. R Foundation for Statistical Computing, Vienna, Austria. Available online: https://cran.r-project.org (accessed on 3 June 2023).
18. Faul, F.; Erdfelder, E.; Lang, A.-G.; Buchner, A. G*Power 3: A flexible statistical power analysis program for the social, behavioral, and biomedical sciences. *Behav. Res. Methods* **2007**, *39*, 175–191. [CrossRef] [PubMed]

19. Julien-Marsollier, F.; Michelet, D.; Assaker, R.; Doval, A.; Louisy, S.; Madre, C.; Simon, A.; Ilharreborde, B.; Brasher, C.; Dahmani, S. Enhanced recovery after surgical correction of adolescent idiopathic scoliosis. *Pediatr. Anesth.* **2020**, *30*, 1068–1076. [CrossRef] [PubMed]
20. Jeandel, C.; Ikonomoff, T.; Bertoncelli, C.M.; Bertoncelli, C.M.; Cunsolo, L.L.; Luna, M.V.; Monticone, M.; Clement, J.-L.; Rampal, V.; Solla, F. Enhanced recovery following posterior spinal fusion for adolescent idiopathic scoliosis: A medical and economic study in a French private nonprofit pediatric hospital. *Orthop Traumatol Surg Res.* **2023**, 103626. [CrossRef]
21. Murphy, R.F.; Mooney, J.F., 3rd. Complications following spine fusion for adolescent idiopathic scoliosis. *Curr. Rev. Musculoskelet. Med.* **2016**, *9*, 462–469. [CrossRef]
22. Levin, D.; Strantzas, S.; Steinberg, B. Intraoperative neuromonitoring in paediatric spinal surgery. *BJA Educ.* **2019**, *19*, 165–171. [CrossRef] [PubMed]
23. Halvorsen, S.; Mehilli, J.; Cassese, S.; Hall, T.S.; Abdelhamid, M.; Barbato, E.; De Hert, S.; de Laval, I.; Geisler, T.; Hinterbuchner, L.; et al. 2022 ESC Guidelines on cardiovascular assessment and management of patients undergoing non-cardiac surgery. *Eur. Heart J.* **2022**, *43*, 3826–3924. [CrossRef] [PubMed]

Disclaimer/Publisher's Note: The statements, opinions and data contained in all publications are solely those of the individual author(s) and contributor(s) and not of MDPI and/or the editor(s). MDPI and/or the editor(s) disclaim responsibility for any injury to people or property resulting from any ideas, methods, instructions or products referred to in the content.

MDPI
St. Alban-Anlage 66
4052 Basel
Switzerland
www.mdpi.com

Children Editorial Office
E-mail: children@mdpi.com
www.mdpi.com/journal/children

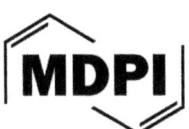

Disclaimer/Publisher's Note: The statements, opinions and data contained in all publications are solely those of the individual author(s) and contributor(s) and not of MDPI and/or the editor(s). MDPI and/or the editor(s) disclaim responsibility for any injury to people or property resulting from any ideas, methods, instructions or products referred to in the content.

www.ingramcontent.com/pod-product-compliance
Lightning Source LLC
LaVergne TN
LVHW070559100526
838202LV00012B/511